Praise for Empowered Mama

"With the most genuine frankness, Ana boils down all things baby-hood and motherhood. Steeped in her experience, sense of humor, and unique sensibility, this book is the gold standard of guides, one which you'll return to baby after baby."

—Annie, homemaker and mom of two

"Ana is like the older sister I never had! As a new mom, I found that Ana's book has been invaluable in the way I have adapted to and approached motherhood. Her practical tips, techniques, and advice are fused in the ways my husband and I raise our son. I have no doubt that we're getting more sleep and our baby is calmer because of the methods we learned from her deep motherly insight and extensive experience. She puts it all on the table and leaves nothing to ponder. This book acts like a loving handholding through parenthood, and I know I'm a more confident mother for it!"

—Maria, new mother

EMPOWERED
Mama

The Real-Talk Guide to Pregnancy, Postpartum Life, and Newborn Care

Ana Hernández Kent, Ph.D.

Empowered Mama
The Real-Talk Guide to Pregnancy, Postpartum Life, and Newborn Care
Ana Hernández Kent, Ph.D.

Published by Trinity House Publishing, St. Louis, MO
Copyright ©2024 Ana Hernández Kent, Ph.D.
All rights reserved.

Project Management and Book Design: Davis Creative Publishing, LLC, DavisCreativePublishing.com
Editor/Proofreader : Carolina VonKampen

Library of Congress Cataloging-in-Publication Data
(Provided by Cassidy Cataloguing Services, Inc.)
Names: Hernández Kent, Ana, author.
Title: Empowered mama : the real-talk guide to pregnancy, postpartum life, and newborn care / Ana Hernández Kent, Ph.D.
Description: St. Louis, MO : Trinity House Publishing, [2024] | Includes bibliographical references.
Identifiers: ISBN: 979-8-9907546-0-7 (paperback) | 979-8-9907546-1-4 (ebook) | LCCN: 2024910136
Subjects: LCSH: Motherhood. | Pregnancy. | Newborn infants--Care. | Postnatal care. | Childbirth. | BISAC: HEALTH & FITNESS / Pregnancy & Childbirth. | FAMILY & RELATIONSHIPS / Life Stages / Infants & Toddlers. | FAMILY & RELATIONSHIPS / Parenting / Motherhood.
Classification: LCC: HQ759 .H47 2024 | DDC: 306.8743--dc23

Dedication

To my three beautiful children.
I couldn't have written this without
the experiences you gave me.
I thank God for the privilege
of being your mother.

And to my husband.
Parenthood is a wild ride.
I'm so blessed and grateful to
have you by my side.
You are my rock and my home.

Table of Contents

Disclaimer

The product information and advice provided in this book are intended for general informational purposes only. The author and publisher of this book have made every effort to ensure that the content is accurate and up-to-date at the time of publication. However, they make no representations or warranties of any kind, express or implied, about the completeness, accuracy, reliability, suitability, or availability of the information, products, or services contained in this book for any purpose.

Preface

Hi there! Congratulations on your pregnancy! There's a lot of newness going on, and while it's exciting, it can also be overwhelming. This book focuses on pregnancy, labor, and the first three months after birth (also known as the fourth trimester): postpartum wellness for you and newborn life for your baby. It gives a real, raw account of what you need to know so that you can feel empowered as a mother.

I set out to write this when my sister-in-law and cousin got pregnant with their first babies around the same time. It was meant to be a short guide to help them, but it quickly turned into something much longer. If you don't have time for the whole thing, don't worry! Read the sections that apply to your needs or skim "The Quick and Dirty Summary" at the end of the book; it won't hurt my feelings.

This guide is based on my experiences being pregnant, going through labor, and raising three kids. Hopefully, this book makes things a little easier for you and helps you understand what to expect. As a researcher, when I got pregnant, I spent hours reading books, articles, and blogs on motherhood, and I read countless reviews and product comparisons while building my baby registry. While fun at times, it can also be exhausting and overwhelming, and we have enough of that going on with all the hormones and later sleep deprivation.

Babies really don't need much—above all, calm and loving parents. This book goes through things grouped by category. Some categories you may choose to ignore because you have experience there, while others might be surprising to you. I'll write a bit about my experience, products I love and some I dislike, and general tips. I won't pretend to be an expert on your child, but I do have three kids and am an "expert" on them—and soon you will be on yours too! Your pregnancy and motherhood journey will no doubt be different from mine, but I hope that this guide is helpful. I'm so excited for you and grateful you've let me share my knowledge.

My motherhood model is simple: give yourself grace. I'm a big proponent of doing what you need to do in order to survive in the moment. At the same time, I hope this book gives you the knowledge and confidence you need to tap into your own strength and move from just surviving to thriving. You've got this, mama.

Love,

Ana

1

Pregnancy:
The Good and the Bad

"Everything grows rounder and wider and weirder, and I sit here in the middle of it all and wonder who in the world you will turn out to be."
—Carrie Fisher

You're pregnant! Congratulations. Pregnancy is unique for every mom, and it can even be different from one pregnancy to the next. Personally, I have mostly hated being pregnant. I'm uncomfortable, nauseous, not as physically able to rely on myself or my body as usual; there's a restricted diet, and I'm miserable much of the time. I'm also extremely tired and bloated, have sore boobs, and, oh, you have to deal with these symptoms without much sympathy at first unless you choose to tell people during the first trimester.

So… what's the good news? Well, first of all, you're pregnant! Your family is growing, and you have a little baby growing inside of you. You are Mother Nature personified—a goddess of life and beauty. It may not always feel that way to you, but you are!

My favorite parts of being pregnant were knowing a sweet little baby was on the way, feeling them kick and move about, and… well that's about it, but it's enough.

First Trimester

Yay, baby! You'll likely have an ultrasound to confirm the pregnancy and hear the baby's heartbeat—an incredible sound. There are a lot of symptoms around this time, like nausea and vomiting. I took prescription medicine for each pregnancy. With my third, the nausea was a lot worse, so I got different medication and a nausea patch, like the type you might use for seasickness. This helped but certainly didn't make the nausea go away completely. It's tough to work with these symptoms; talk to your boss in confidence if you need accommodations at work.

There's also a heightened sense of smell, as in, everything stinks and makes you nauseous, and you feel like a damn bloodhound. I had to completely avoid the space 50 feet from my work's cafeteria for months or hold my breath as much as possible while I grabbed a quick lunch. If you have favorite products—shampoos, soaps, deodorant, mouthwash, etc.—I highly recommend choosing different products to use during your pregnancy. Seriously. There are soaps I no longer use because I still associate them with nausea; I also threw away my husband's Listerine, and he knows he is no longer allowed to buy that flavor.

What helps with the nausea? Prescription medicine, but I also found that eating smaller meals throughout the day helped as well—never being too hungry or too full. Ginger and lemon supposedly help, though not really in my experience. Eating an omelet in the morning has also helped me; perhaps it's the protein? Stay hydrated! This is especially true if you're vomiting. If water is no longer appealing to you, try flavoring it with fruit. Having regular bowel movements can also help, strange as that may sound (my doctor told me this first, and I've found that it's true). Use a stool softener if you're having trouble having a bowel movement (constipation can be common too).

During this trimester, you'll also be more tired than you've ever been. Lean into this, especially your first pregnancy when you don't have other kids and can actually rest. Your body is growing an entire human, and it needs that extra rest and sleep. Go to bed early, sleep in late (you won't be able to for the next decade or so, so enjoy it while you can), and nap too. Invest in a pregnancy pillow. It's especially nice to have later on in your third trimester. My husband is jealous every time

I pull mine out, which is the U-shaped kind that I place upside down. It helps with pains later on in pregnancy too. One other side effect of being pregnant: your boobs may hurt and grow; mine never did too badly, but it's common.

Also, this trimester you will be given the option for genetic screening and to find out the sex of the baby. We didn't do this screening for any baby. While usually I'm a firm believer that knowledge is power, it wouldn't change my decision to have the baby, so in this case we didn't do it. As for knowing the sex, we didn't with my first baby because we wanted to be surprised. With the next two, our lives were already chaotic, so we wanted to know and have the name prepared (we had a hard time picking a second boy name).

Importantly, take a prenatal vitamin every day. Ideally, you'll have been taking these since before you even knew you were pregnant. If you haven't been, start today. I've used several different kinds, including One A Day, but my current favorite is Ritual, which tells you where they source each ingredient and has a not-too-strong citrus flavor. You'll also take these after you give birth if you breastfeed, so pick one you like!

Surprised by how much you have to pee? It's the hormones. Stay hydrated even though these frequent bathroom trips are annoying.

One more thing: If you're planning on going back to work, you should immediately put your child on a daycare wait list (or start looking for a nanny). Wait lists can be longer than your pregnancy! With my second child, I didn't tell daycare until I was about four months pregnant, and we didn't get a spot until four months after I needed it. With my third child, our daycare knew I was pregnant before we even told my parents.

By the way, in 2022, the Pregnant Workers Fairness Act went into effect. It mandates reasonable accommodations for pregnant workers unless providing them would impose an undue hardship on their employer. So, don't be afraid to ask for what you need from your employer, especially if you have a doctor's note.

Second Trimester

The second trimester is known as the honeymoon trimester. Your terrible first trimester symptoms may lessen or go away entirely. For me, the nausea with my third child, which was the worst of all three, lasted throughout the second trimester, though the vomiting slowed down. During this trimester, you'll feel your baby move for the first time, and you'll have more energy. You'll also likely tell people about the pregnancy more broadly and start showing, but in a cute way, earning you many compliments. There's no "right" time to share the news, but waiting until the end of the first trimester is a good rule of thumb.

Because you're past some of the yucky symptoms and you haven't gotten to feeling like a bloated walrus in the third trimester, take advantage! Go out to fancy dinners and take a babymoon if you can. It's good to focus on your relationship with your partner before you're both focused on keeping a tiny human alive.

It's also a good time to take a newborn and/or labor class if you're interested. These are typically offered by your hospital and are good for expecting new parents. Grandparent and sibling classes are sometimes offered as well, but these aren't really necessary. You can also research and pick a pediatrician during this trimester. You'll want to be comfortable with that person—do they listen to your concerns in a compassionate and nondismissive way? Is the location easy to get to (you'll be there a lot)? How quickly can your child be seen for sick visits? What is the vaccination schedule like? Are there multiple pediatricians at the practice so your child can be seen even when their usual doctor is sick or on vacation? It's an important decision, so don't put it off until later.

During the second trimester, you'll do the glucose screening, which means you'll drink a sugary drink that really doesn't taste too bad, wait an hour, and have blood drawn. I never tested positive for gestational diabetes, thankfully, but work with your doctor if you do.

One of the most exciting parts of pregnancy for me was feeling the baby. For my first, I was about 20 weeks along when I felt a little flutter while I was at church. I knew immediately what it was. For my subsequent pregnancies, I felt it sooner—around 15 to 16 weeks. The baby's little flutters soon become potent elbows and kicks, along with the occasional hiccup. It's really amazing—a way that you can feel your baby that no one else can. By the third trimester, others can feel it too (though in a different way). Plus, you can actually see your baby moving sometimes in your belly, which is weird but also neat. They tend to move a bit more at night when you're still, and less during the day because your movement is soothing and puts them in a sleepier state. This is also why many babies confuse night and day when they're newborns.

Ask your doctor about getting vaccinated for certain things. You'll need a Tdap vaccine each pregnancy, but there are others you should consider too. Getting immunized while you're pregnant can pass some of those benefits along to your fetus. This is especially great if your baby will be born in the winter. For example, your baby can't get the flu or COVID-19 vaccines until they're at least six months old, but you can get those vaccines while you're pregnant with your baby, and that will help give them some protection. If you get immunized while breastfeeding, you'll pass along some of those benefits to the baby as well.

Speaking of vaccinations, ask your baby's inner circle—those that will be physically closest to the baby and holding them those first two months—to check on their Tdap immunizations. They should have had one in the past 10 years. If not, ask that they update it. It's ultimately their choice, but it's *your* choice whether or not to let them around your baby when they are young and vulnerable. As a parent, one of your main jobs is to speak up for your child when they can't do it themselves, and that means having uncomfortable conversations or even upsetting people close to you when necessary. People may disagree with you, but if they don't respect your wishes and the way you're bringing up your child, it's okay to politely and firmly stick to your guns.

Third Trimester

The "I'm huge/get this baby out of me" trimester. I didn't really experience the latter, but I certainly felt huge, particularly with the second and third babies. There's some tiredness again and swelling of the hands and feet. Some women have to take off their wedding rings because their fingers swell so much, though I was able to keep mine on throughout the entire pregnancy. Comfortable shoes are a must, as is ease of putting them on (think slip-on, no laces). You can size up or go for wider shoes. You may have heard that your feet can grow a half or full size, and this lengthening sticks around after pregnancy. I found that this did happen to me, especially after the second and third babies (the half size up is in total, not for each pregnancy, thankfully!). What I didn't know was why, at least not until I went in to get new ski boots because my feet were in so much pain. The man attending me knew the reason—because your feet flatten a bit; they don't actually grow. The arch just flattens, causing your foot to get longer. Who knew?

This is also the trimester that can be an emotionally hard pill to swallow in terms of asking for help. I've always been highly independent, but I believe pregnancy is uniquely designed by God to slow us down gradually so the newborn months (also known as the fourth trimester) are not as much of a shock to our lifestyles. Ask for help lifting things. Accept that you won't walk as quickly and even going up a flight of stairs can wind you (the baby is taking up tons of room in there, squishing your lungs and bladder). Stay hydrated, especially if you're in this trimester during the summer months, as I was with my first two babies. I almost passed out from getting overheated once, and that was a scary experience I'd not care to repeat. Take advantage of floating in a pool if you can. It takes the weight off your aching feet and feels really good. Set up the nursery and pack your hospital bag a month out so you don't have to worry about it later (see chapter 2 for a hospital packing list).

Also, accept that you will use the bathroom every hour or so. The baby is now putting pressure on your bladder (you can tell because it may lighten or get worse as they change position). This is incredibly annoying but par for the course. Don't limit water intake to attempt to not pee so frequently; it doesn't work and will just leave you dehydrated. Try to pee again after you just stopped; you'll probably get a bit more out. You can also lean forward and try peeing more. Another tip: pee right before getting in the car, no matter where you are going or how recently you had peed before this. I've definitely been in a situation where I thought I could make it through my 30-minute commute, only to realize I couldn't and had to stop at a random building and beg to use their restroom. You may feel fine, but then the baby decides to tap dance on your bladder. Moral of the story—always pee when you can.

You'll also have more tests this trimester. I tested positive for GBS bacteria (Group B strep) with my second two babies. It's not a big deal and it's very common; you just get two rounds of antibiotics during labor. I only got one with each because my labors were so fast, and that's fine too. Passing it on to your baby is very rare, even without the antibiotics (but still get them if you test positive!).

One additional nasty symptom I've experienced starting in my third trimester with my second baby, and in my second trimester with my third, is pubic symphysis pain. A great pregnancy and postpartum fitness guru, Abby Erker, identified this immediately when I explained my symptoms. Your pelvis is relaxing and loosening up to make room for the baby during birth, but this means that there can be some pain in your pelvic area. For me, it was fairly centrally located on my pubic bone. The pain usually flared up when walking or even standing for longer periods of time, and it was no fun. Strangely, during a trip to London, we were walking several miles each day, and this actually seemed to help lessen the pain. The good thing is the pubic symphysis pain usually goes away after labor (though for my first baby it only showed up *after* labor).

Eliminating asymmetrical movements (think squats on one leg, getting out of the car with one leg first, rolling over in bed with your legs separating) is key. Keep your legs together as much as you can. A pelvic floor therapist recommended pretending you're in a pencil skirt all the time. You might also try a maternity support band or even athletic tape on your belly to help support the extra weight. You can look up pelvic floor exercises online or go to a pelvic floor physical therapist if you need more tips.

Finally, try to mentally prepare yourself for labor and newborn life. Accept that your lifestyle and your body will change, and that's a beautiful thing.

Maternity Clothes

I hate maternity clothes, but they're a necessary evil. They almost never look cute, and they're surprisingly expensive. Yet it makes sense to invest in several pieces, especially if you plan on having more than one baby. Your first pregnancy, you most likely won't need to stop wearing your normal clothes until the end of the second or even the third trimester. That's especially true for clothes with more give or room, like yoga pants and flowy shirts and dresses. Betabrand has dress pant yoga pants (they're thick and don't look like yoga pants at all). They're not maternity-specific, but with the stretchiness, I find I can wear them for a long time through the second trimester.

I suggest getting a few maternity dresses, pants, yoga pants, and tops. You can also borrow your husband's or partner's bigger shirts for a bit (it's the least they can do for getting you in this situation). Ingrid & Isabel is sold by Target and has decent maternity clothes. Old Navy maternity clothes are also not bad. In general, when buying maternity pants, I recommend opting for the full-panel ones. These grow the best with you, don't cut in like half-panel ones, and last longer than the side-panel ones (really only good for the second trimester).

Maternity underwear is terrible. All the brands I've tried are incredibly low-cut, with an overlapping V shape in the middle front. When I say low-cut, I mean sitting well below the natural hairline—just not comfortable. I admit I have a voluptuous backside, though I imagine these would be uncomfortable for many women. Perhaps they were designed by men? Anyway, I suggest sizing up on your regular, breathable underwear. Speaking of, you may want to regularly wear a panty liner if you don't already because you may experience more discharge during pregnancy than you normally do.

As for bras, you can continue wearing your normal one, but if that's uncomfortable, I suggest buying nursing bras. That way you can use them after pregnancy too (if you choose to breastfeed). Most of them don't have underwire, and you can get a size that fits your larger breasts. There are two kinds: the ones that have a clip on each side, allowing you to unclip and lower the panel to nurse (a smaller side panel behind the main one attaches to the strap), and the ones that are more like a V where you just slip your breast out. Both are just okay, though I prefer the former because I find they hold my breasts in better (as a C/D cup). There are also nursing camisoles, which are nice when you're out in public because your midriff will never be exposed while nursing.

Ultrasounds

You will get a few ultrasounds. I had one to confirm the pregnancy, the long anatomy one at 20 weeks, and one later in the third trimester. Sometimes your doctor will want more, and sometimes less. There are also places you can go to and pay for three-dimensional ultrasounds and pictures if your doctor doesn't offer that (mine did with my third child). I did the three-dimensional ultrasound with my first baby. I had to go twice because he didn't cooperate the first time (or the second) and hid his little face. I'd say in the end it's a personal choice but not truly worth it. While exciting and cute, these pictures don't do justice to your newborn baby's beautiful face.

Diet

Your life is no longer just your own, and one of the first ways you experience this is through a restricted pregnancy diet. You may have food aversions and cravings. Adjust to these, and let others know about them as well.

For instance, during my second pregnancy, I was trapped on a two-hour flight with my family, who had chosen to bring barbecue on the plane for dinner. I couldn't stand the smell, and it was awful. Luckily, since it was about a year after the COVID-19 pandemic, an aunt had masks in her purse, and I wore a double mask for the duration of the flight to block out the smell.

There are many lists out there about what to avoid, so I won't go into too much detail. Some are obvious (alcohol), while others (certain types of fish) are not. Generally, unpasteurized foods (juices, cheeses, etc.) are off-limits, as are raw meats and fish, lunch meats, and sprouts. You should also stay away from prepared cold salads, like tuna and chicken salad, that have been sitting out. It's fine to prepare these for yourself at home. Chick-fil-A lemonade is not pasteurized, so it's best to stay away from it (I'm pointing this one out specifically because I see this question frequently on pregnancy forums).

I've heard people think that honey is off-limits; it's not for pregnant people, but it *is* for infants under age one. Caffeine should be limited. With my first, I didn't do any caffeine at all. By the third, I had one 8-to-12-ounce coffee a day. Not every day, but many days. When in doubt, ask your doctor.

There are ways to get around some of the above. For example, I don't love cold cuts normally, but when I'm pregnant, I really want them. It may have something to do with the fact that I can't have them. To appease my craving, I heat up the lunch meat on a stovetop until steaming. This is supposed to kill any possible listeria bacteria (the reason you shouldn't eat it cold). If you're craving sushi, you can try cooked sushi, like shrimp tempura or unagi (eel, which is poisonous when uncooked so it's always cooked). Small amounts of caffeine can help when you're really dragging, as I already mentioned. Risks from the above are generally small, but your baby is also small, so why risk it?

If you're wondering if you can really "eat for two", the answer is not exactly, at least not like an additional adult. The amount of extra fuel you need depends on a few factors, like your prepregnancy weight, your activity level, and your metabolism. The general guidelines are something like zero to 50 extra calories per day during your first trimester, 200 to 350 during your second trimester, and about 450 during your third trimester. My suggestion is don't stress too much about it and just have some healthy snacks on hand that are palatable to you.

Environment

Speaking of risks, the smaller your baby, the greater the risks of teratogens. These are things in your environment (like smoke) or things you ingest that can cause fetal abnormalities. Use common sense. Don't use drugs, drink, smoke, or be around others who smoke (cigarettes, cigars, marijuana, etc.). Ask your doctor before taking medications. For example, acetaminophen (e.g., Tylenol) is fine, while ibuprofen (e.g., Advil, Motrin) is not.

You may also consider cutting plastics from your life. For example, use glass containers or porcelain plates, especially when reheating in the microwave. Because of the fumes, I also refused to paint my nails or paint while pregnant (though I did paint a safari mural in the nursery while pregnant with my first; I just kept the windows and doors open).

Speaking of fumes, with my first baby I made my husband pump my car's gasoline every time so that I wouldn't inhale the fumes. I don't strictly think this is necessary (and I pumped my own gas with my third), but it's worth mentioning. The point is that you should think about your environment—what you're putting in or on your body and what you're surrounded by—and how that could affect your tiny baby.

Some women wonder about hot tubs and baths. Hot tubs are out, but warm baths and showers are okay. Your skin shouldn't feel hot or be red when you get out of the bath or shower. The main thing is you don't want to raise your body temperature too much.

Travel

Take a babymoon if you can! Once you get farther along (past 36 weeks), it's a good idea to limit travel—plane travel especially because of swelling and the possibility of developing a blood clot, but long car travel as well. If you must travel, then stop along the way to stretch your legs and stay hydrated. You'll probably have to stop every hour or so to pee anyway.

I went to London for a last-hurrah vacation with my husband and our two kids when I was 34 weeks pregnant with our third. Technically, they say to limit international travel after 28 weeks, but I didn't know this when booking the trip (and likely wouldn't have cared). It all worked out for me, but the baby can definitely come early, so maybe don't cut it as close as I did! Tell your doctor about travel plans in the third trimester and research hospitals at your destination just in case.

Miscarriage

This is a sad topic, and it's one that is scary, but it is *incredibly common.* Miscarriage is when the pregnancy is lost before 20 weeks. Studies estimate that between 10–20 percent of known pregnancies end in miscarriage. That doesn't include unknown pregnancies. I had no idea about this because in our society it's not discussed.

I had a miscarriage before my firstborn baby. I was six weeks along, and it was devastating. I don't talk about it—ever—or at least I haven't except to close family and friends who were going through something similar. I'm writing about it now, even though it's scary to reveal so much of myself personally and it still hurts to think and talk about, because I hope that it can help even just one mom who has been shattered by the same thing.

What helped me get through this time was therapy. My therapist shared her own story of miscarriage, which was by far the most helpful thing to me going through it, and it's why I'm sharing my story here. She said that she had similar feelings (of sadness and anger), but if she hadn't had that miscarriage, she never would have gotten pregnant with her now 20-something-year-old twins, and she couldn't imagine life without them. This really stuck with me. Sure enough, three months later I was pregnant with David, my firstborn.

The emotional pain of the miscarriage is still there, but there is reluctant acceptance as well. Especially when I learned most miscarriages are due to chromosome malformation, I accepted that I wouldn't want to bring a child into the world that experienced significant health problems and pain, for their sake.

I will say that my miscarriage affected my feelings toward my second pregnancy a lot, particularly the first trimester. I didn't take a pregnancy test and only went to the doctor for an ultrasound when it was clear I had missed two periods. At the ultrasound, we heard the heartbeat, and I couldn't even smile. I just felt terror—fear that it would happen again. (By the way, once the heartbeat is heard, chances of a miscarriage decrease significantly, but I was still afraid.) Sometimes I think women were better off a century ago when there weren't early-detection pregnancy tests and ultrasounds, because many of those miscarriages would likely have been attributed to a late period. I've skipped periods in the past, so I probably would have thought it was the same with my miscarriage had I not known I was pregnant.

That fear has lingered in some way for all of my pregnancies until the time the babies are born. And then it's replaced by worry about their safety as a newborn, toddler, and child. So, I suppose that worry is always part of being a mother. Some amount of worry is normal.

If you are going through a miscarriage, a stillbirth (when the baby dies in the womb after 20 weeks of pregnancy), or are having trouble conceiving, my heart goes out to you. Talk to someone, anyone, and know that you are not alone.

2

Labor and Hospital Stay

"When you feel like you can't and you do,
that's when you find your power."

—Camila Ramón, Peloton cycling instructor

*L*abor is… nerve-racking. No doubt you've seen labors in TV shows or movies, but what is it really like?

I was dreading labor with my first baby. Not knowing what to expect, other than a lot of pain, was very worrisome. Of course, women all over the world have done it since the dawn of time, but that doesn't mean it's not scary.

What (and When) to Pack

I suggest packing your hospital bag a month before your due date. Nag your significant other to pack theirs as well, otherwise they will be frantically throwing things in a bag while you're in labor and waiting to go to the hospital, like mine was with our third baby when I went into labor a week early.

So, what do you need? The following are just suggestions, but I've found them useful.

- ID and insurance cards.
- Robe. You'll have mesh underwear on at the hospital, and you'll need easy access to your breasts to nurse if you're breastfeeding. I wore a short, breathable robe for two days after each of my labors.

- Phone and charger. Pack one if you have a spare so that you don't forget later. Also, put your phone on Do Not Disturb mode immediately after getting to the hospital (and don't remove that setting for the first few months, at least). Answer calls and texts on your own time. As a bonus, you can add certain people (like your significant other) as favorites, and this allows them to bypass this setting.
- Toothbrush and toothpaste. I just threw in a disposable one that you get from the dentist (we have a stockpile) and a travel-sized toothpaste.
- Shampoo, conditioner, and soap. The hospital will provide soap, but it can be nice to have your own brand for that first shower. Plus, they may not give you shampoo or conditioner (mine didn't), so pack a travel-sized one of each of those.
- Prenatal vitamins. The hospital will provide these too, but it's nice to have your own brand. You will continue taking these if you decide to breastfeed. You can also take a postnatal vitamin instead (Ritual offers one).
- Contacts or glasses if you wear them.
- Slippers. Unless you want to walk barefoot on the cold hospital floor, I suggest packing a pair.
- Heating pad. This really helped me with labor pain when pressed onto my lower back.
- Going home outfit for your baby. With my first son, we packed the cutest pants with suspenders and a button-down shirt. It was a mistake. It's hard to get babies dressed, particularly when they're so young. Plus, it wasn't soft or comfortable. For our second son, I packed a long-sleeve sleeper/footie personalized with his name and a matching monogrammed hat (which I got off of Etsy). Still super cute but infinitely more comfortable and easier to put him in.

- Going home outfit for you. Pack something easy to wear, and maybe skip the pants unless it's cold outside. I just packed a soft maternity dress that was nursing friendly. You might also want a nursing bra or two.
- Pajamas. I usually packed two of my husband's shirts and walked around without bottoms, other than the horrid (but necessary) mesh underwear. Pack whatever is comfortable for you.
- Pillow. You might want to pack your own pillow. The hospital ones are very thin.
- Nursing pillow. You can use a hospital pillow instead, but if you have room, a nursing pillow can be more comfortable, especially while you're learning how to breastfeed your newborn.
- Your own ice pack pads. This isn't necessary at all because the hospital will provide you with some, but if you purchased these, your time in the hospital is likely when you'll be using them.
- Light makeup. The first time I read this suggestion, the feminist in me found it completely ridiculous. But then I wished I had some with me for the newborn pictures in the hospital the next day (not during labor; everything will sweat off anyway). Nothing over the top—just a little mascara and lip gloss. It's a personal choice, but if it makes you happier looking back on those first few photos, then why not?
- Entertainment. Personally, I don't think you need to pack this. There isn't a ton of downtime, and you're focused on giving birth. Plus, your phone can probably provide entertainment if there is a lull. But if it you have room, you might pack a book or something small to pass the time.

The hospital will provide much of what you and your baby need. They will likely give you mesh underwear, humongous pads, a peri bottle, witch hazel pads (probably Tucks), ice packs, medication, and the bare necessities for showering and sleeping. For your baby, they will have swaddles, hats, diapers, and wipes.

Am I in Labor?

So, what does it feel like, and how will you know you're in labor? Basically, it feels like concentrated, intense period cramps. This was a bit surprising to me because for some reason, I expected the pain to be more evenly distributed throughout my body. It was not. It wraps around your lower stomach. Some women also experience intense back pain, which I did not. Labor, as I said, basically feels like menstrual cramps but quite a bit worse. You'll know it's the "real" thing (as opposed to Braxton Hicks, or practice, contractions) because the cramps do not lessen and instead become more frequent and more intense. They're not too bad in the beginning. You should follow the 4-1-1 rule: Go to the hospital when your contractions are four minutes apart, one minute in duration, for at least one hour, or if you're in doubt or believe something is wrong.

With my first, I started feeling something around 9 a.m., but it was very infrequent. By 9 p.m., my contractions were closer to the 4-1-1 rule, and we went to the hospital. My son was born eight hours later. I went into labor on his due date. With my second baby, I went into labor three days after my due date, and I had tried acupuncture, long walks, and squats a few days leading up to labor because I didn't want to have to be induced. We were in the hospital around five hours with her. With my third, I had been feeling mild contractions all day but knew this would be the last few moments of relative freedom, so I ignored them as long as I could. We got to the hospital around 8 p.m. at four centimeters dilated, and he was born three hours later. Despite him being sunny-side up, it was a quick and easy labor.

A note about Braxton Hicks contractions: some women have them and some don't. I didn't with my first, but each subsequent pregnancy I have felt them more and more. They're not really painful and go away quickly.

Labor

The most important thing about a birth plan is that it should be flexible. You never know how you're going to feel in the moment or if something might necessitate a change.

With all three babies I had a vaginal birth. My first birth, I wanted to do a natural, unmedicated birth, or at least start out that way. After a few hours with increasingly painful contractions, I remember saying to the nurse, "Even though there's a lot of individual variability, roughly how much longer?" She basically said there was no way to tell. I was about seven centimeters dilated at the time, and I knew it could go on for many more hours, so I asked for an epidural. I believe that was a good call. It took about an hour for the epidural technician to get to me, and by that time I was having contractions that, in my words, had gone from "red" pain to "black" pain. Certainly, it was the most pain I had experienced in my life. I'm glad I didn't continue on unmedicated through active labor. I will say that the pain did not go away completely, and you can control additional doses of pain medicine. With my first and second babies, I still definitely felt a good amount of pain even with the epidurals. With my third, I did not, so I suppose it just depends on the epidural.

Also, with each birth, I had my waters broken at the hospital. I was worried I would have my water embarrassingly break at work, so I'm very glad this didn't happen. Each baby came quickly after that—my second baby within 15 minutes after my water breaking. She was so fast, in fact, that between the time I felt intense pressure and yelled at my husband to get help, the poor nurse barely had time to run into the room before the baby was out.

A few additional notes on the epidural: I got mine while sitting up, but some epidurals are given while you're lying down. They numb the spot on your mid to lower back, which feels like a big pinch, and then they give you the pain medicine. You stay hooked up to the medicine so you can give yourself more as needed. You need to stay perfectly still for the insertion, even if you're having contractions. My third time, the epidural insertion site was incredibly itchy for the next day or so; it's a common side effect. I was also extremely cold after the birth, to the point of shivering. This only happened with my third labor. Finally, after they give you the epidural, your legs are mostly numb, so you can't walk around for the rest of your labor and have to stay in bed, which is something to keep in mind. Also, you'll be given a catheter. This doesn't hurt since you'll already be numb, but it's necessary because you won't know if you have to pee or not.

Talking about the bathroom, you may have heard that you will poop when you give birth. This is true for many women, and it happens because pushing at the end of labor is a bearing down that feels exactly like pooping. Don't hold back, or you will make labor much harder for yourself (and your baby). The medical staff is used to it; if it happens, they will simply clean it up. I'll note that I did not poop with my first or second (I didn't ask with my third baby). I think it's because with my first, I labored naturally for a while and had several bowel movements (in the toilet) because the baby was moving down to the birth canal and literally pushing everything out. I also had a bowel movement at the beginning of labor with my second. It's one of the signs that labor is coming soon, and it's your body's way of preparing and making room.

My first birth was vacuum-assisted, meaning they put a suction device on the baby's head while in utero and then use gentle suction to help get him out. It was necessary because his heart rate dropped a bit. With all three labors, I had a first-degree laceration (the least intense) requiring stitches. These stitches dissolve by themselves and can be a bit itchy.

After the birth with my first, I felt as if a semitruck had hit me. I was exhausted and in some pain but mostly sore. By the time I had my third, I felt strangely normal after labor. My body was just used to it, I suppose, and it was a much shorter labor.

Many women have labors that are more difficult than mine. I've been lucky. What helped me most was the epidural, heat (I suggest bringing an electronic heating pad), and water (during the first birth, I was in a tub much of the time before I chose the epidural). Each birth is unique, and no, it is not a pleasant experience, but the pain is short-lived and your baby is for the rest of your life.

One more thing: This is the time to do cord blood banking and/or tissue collection if you want. I've done it with all three. You sign up with a service (I use Cord Blood Registry), and they send you a kit. You fill out some information before the birth and make sure your nurse and doctor know at the beginning of your labor that you would like the cord blood or tissue collected. The sample is collected after the birth and doesn't hurt you or your baby. Then, you call a courier service to immediately pick it up. I suggest you assign this task to your significant other; you will have enough on your mind. That being said, mine forgot the last time and I had to call—luckily, I remembered within the time limit.

The pros of cord blood banking are that the service stores this blood, which can supposedly be used in the future in case your child or a sibling gets seriously ill, and it's supposed to be effective because it's a perfect genetic match. The cons are that it's very expensive, and the companies charge a yearly maintenance fee (unless you sign up for a lifetime plan). In all likelihood, your child will never need or benefit from this storage. However, since we could afford it, my family chose to store the cord blood. It's a personal choice. Do your research to see if cord blood storage is right for you.

Some hospitals give you the option to donate your cord blood to be banked. This is free, but the blood can be used for anyone who needs it, and it won't be "saved" for your child. It's a nice thing to do, although my hospital no longer offers this and yours may or may not.

After Labor

Right after birth, you can decide whether or not you want the medical staff to hold off on some tests on your baby so you can have an hour of skin-to-skin (highly recommend) and breastfeed if that's what you want to do (see chapter 5 on breastfeeding for tips). You'll probably also be asked if you want your baby to have antibiotic eye drops and a vitamin K shot. These are standard and can prevent issues later. Your baby will also be evaluated for an Apgar score to see if they need more intense care, and they'll have a hearing test about 24 hours after birth.

Skin-to-skin time right after birth is a great opportunity to nurse your baby. They might even be rooting around trying to find your nipple. More on this in the breastfeeding chapter, but gently guide their mouths to your nipple. They should open their mouths and you can pull them in to help them latch on.

If your baby is a boy, you'll be asked whether or not you want to circumcise them. I left this decision up to my husband because he's the one with a penis, and he wanted both our boys circumcised. They take the baby away and may give him different things for the pain, including sugar, Tylenol, a pacifier, and a numbing agent. I really struggled with this because I didn't want him to be in pain. Other than the crying I'm sure each son did when the procedure was conducted, both boys were mostly just sleepy and didn't cry more often than my daughter over the next day. See chapter 3 on the first two days for more on circumcision care.

Your doctor will sew you up if you've had any tearing, and your nurses will monitor your bleeding and press down on your abdomen. This is called a fundal massage. It's not pleasant, but it helps the uterus contract and prevents postpartum hemorrhaging. You may also experience uterine cramping for a day or two after giving birth, which likewise helps your uterus contract. These cramps were worse with each subsequent birth. Finally, if you've had an epidural, it will be removed, along with the catheter.

You may have people waiting in the delivery area who are dying to meet your sweet baby. You may be okay with this, or you may want to hold off. We had both sets of grandparents and both aunts all come in at the same time, about an hour after the birth, and that was overwhelming, both because I was exhausted and it was a small room. Also, I was pretty emotional after birth and it felt strange to have my baby so far away from me, even though it was only a few feet. My suggestion is to ask your family to wait at home until you call them. That way, you can manage who comes in and when, and you can space out the visitors a bit too. I also recommend you limit hospital visitors to immediate family; everyone else can wait until you're home and settled.

3

Your Baby's Here!
The First Two Days

"Being able to hold my son and see him is awesome."
—Jonathan, my cousin

*T*here's nothing quite like meeting your baby for the first time. That tiny face is perfection, and those 10 little fingers and toes are impossibly small. You might be surprised by how your baby looks. Depending on how long they are in the birth canal, their head might be a little cone-shaped (it will round out), and they may be skinnier than you expect (those rolls, if they come, will likely be put on later). They may look a bit splotchy—the skin is very thin; remember they just went through labor themselves— and they may or may not have hair in unexpected places, like their back or ears (this is called lanugo and is more likely if they are born earlier). You may not really be able to tell what eye color they have, not just because they don't keep them open much in the beginning, but because it changes, even in the first few days after birth. Their skin may also seem a bit wrinkly because they haven't filled out much. In other words, your newborn looks like a newborn, not like a three-month-old infant (chubby, with smooth, soft skin), which is of-tentimes what we expect them to look like. But they are yours, and they are beautiful.

Checking on You and Sleep

I've covered some of the first few hours immediately after labor in the previous chapter's labor section, but after that, what happens? You and your baby will be taken to a different room where you will stay until you are discharged. The nurse will come by several times to check on your bleeding and uterus (doing this by firmly and somewhat painfully pressing down on your abdomen). If you've had an epidural, the nurse will be there the first few times you pee to make sure your legs can support you and you don't collapse. (Although for me, the numbing effects of the epidural have always gone away pretty quickly once it's taken out.) Your doctor will also likely prescribe you pain medication. I suggest taking it as prescribed when in the hospital and then seeing how you feel once you get home and taking it when you're in pain. Don't be a martyr.

What about the baby? Mostly, your baby sleeps. You will likely have the option to room-in with your baby (they sleep in a bassinet on wheels in your room), or you can choose to have them taken to the nursery and brought back to you when it's time to eat, approximately every three hours around the clock. Before I had my first baby, it was recommended to me that I take advantage of the nursery. Having gone through it three times now, I recommend the same to you. With my second, she was born during the late COVID-19 era and there was no nursery option, so I had her in the room with me. Having done both, I can tell you that the nursery option is better (in my opinion). You're able to really rest and sleep when they are in the nursery. The nurses there do this all the time and are pros at taking care of babies. Your baby will be brought back to you when they are hungry, and in the meantime, you can sleep, eat, and shower in peace. You won't be waking up every few minutes because your baby made a noise and you need to make sure they're okay. Babies are *very* loud sleepers (more on this in chapter 4, the sleep chapter). Plus, you'll likely be rooming-in with your newborn very soon; take advantage of the overnight help while you can.

Checking on Your Baby

In addition to several checks on you and your baby, the nurse will ask if you want them to bathe your baby. Your baby will have their hair (if they have any) plastered to their head by the blood and amniotic fluid from birth, and there might be some on their body as well. I prefer to delay the bath for 24 hours to let the baby's body temperature regulate as much as it can. I also like to rub the vernix caseosa (the white stuff on the baby) into the baby's skin so they can get maximum benefit from that great moisturizer. If your baby is born close to full-term, they won't have too much on their body, and babies born earlier will have more. The vernix helps their skin retain moisture and may be associated with helping them latch onto your breast. I do suggest you let the nurse bathe your baby after 24 hours though. This way they are clean when you take them home. Just a head's up: when looking at your naked baby, you might see that their genitals look a bit swollen (both boys and girls). This is normal, and the swelling will decrease on its own after a few days.

If your baby boy is to be circumcised, this will likely happen soon after the birth. (Though it can be delayed, I think it's probably better to get it over with. Talk with your pediatrician about the pros and cons.) Circumcision care starts at the hospital. The tip of the penis will be very red, and you'll need to keep gauze and a heaping ton of petroleum jelly (Vaseline) on it while it heals. You'll change this out during every diaper change for the first week or so. If the gauze gets stuck, *do not pull it off!* This happened with my first son, and the nurse patiently squeezed warm water on the stuck gauze until it released. Be very gentle. To clean, just use warm water; don't use baby wipes. Call your pediatrician if you notice anything that seems off, like blood or signs of infection, or if your baby isn't peeing.

Newborns will have an umbilical cord stump, which will dry out and brown over the next few days. Don't pull on it or attempt to take it off. You don't have to do anything to care for it except keep it dry. Make sure the diaper isn't covering the stump, and don't submerse your baby in water until the stump falls off (within two weeks of birth).

The whites of your baby's eyes may look slightly yellow a few days after birth. This is because of jaundice and is fairly common. If it doesn't go away by their second-week pediatrician visit, their doctor may recommend treatment.

Newborn Photos

Sometime during your hospital stay, you may have a photographer come by asking if you want newborn photos taken. Say yes. With my first, I didn't, reasoning I could do it myself and we were going to have our own photographer do some later. I regret not having them taken at the hospital. Your baby changes so much those first few weeks, even those first few days! Their face and body fill out. They quickly gain weight (though may lose some during the first two weeks) and gain length as well. Plus, the photographer does this several times a day and is a pro at quickly posing your baby (and you with your baby); a session doesn't take more than 15 minutes. You don't need to purchase the photos later, but at least you'll have the option.

Speaking of newborn photos, if you're going to have them done after the hospital too, make sure to do them within the first two weeks, three at the latest. I suggest sometime the second week. Give your photographer a head's up regarding your due date so that you can quickly schedule a session. You want to do it soon after the birth not only because your newborn changes so much, but also because they become significantly less sleepy. If you want those sweet newborn poses (curled up, naked, little head posing with their cute hands, etc.), your best chance at getting those will be in the first three weeks, after the baby is happily fed and sleeping.

Caring for You, Too

There will be more on this in the postpartum care chapter, but don't forget to take care of yourself those first few days. Your emotions are running high, and your body has been through severe physical trauma. Don't forget that, even if you're feeling okay. Rest every minute you can, take a shower when a nurse or your partner can watch the baby (more on shower care in chapter 6 about postpartum care), eat the hospital food (or enlist someone to bring you sushi or a cold-cut sandwich, stat), and drink plenty of water (caffeine can wait or perhaps limit it). Drinking water is especially important if you're breastfeeding. A rule of thumb I've seen is eight ounces per nursing session. I have no trouble meeting this usually because when I breastfeed, I've never been thirstier. Listen to your body.

Other Notes

A few items of business you'll need to take care of. You'll be given some forms to fill out in order to get your baby a birth certificate (this will be sent out about a month after birth) and a social security number. Obviously, these are very important things to do, so don't procrastinate! Enlist your significant other if you can (it's the least they can do!).

If you have an uncomplicated vaginal birth, you'll probably be released from the hospital two days later. If you have a C-section, it might be up to four days later, from what I understand. You'll have to sign a form saying you have a car seat and have it installed properly. When you're discharged, your pediatrician (or the hospital pediatrician if yours doesn't do hospital visits) will check your baby. Then, when you're given the green light, someone will come up and wheel you out to your car in a wheelchair with your baby in your arms. They don't let you walk; it's probably a liability thing.

Visitors

Finally, a quick note on visitors. I've mentioned most of this already, but *you* decide who can see your baby, when they can see your baby, and what they should do before seeing your baby. Ask those in your baby's inner circle to have updated Tdap vaccines, and everyone should wash their hands before touching the baby. I'd also suggest not letting them touch your baby's hands or their face. Our germs are just too big for newborns because they don't have any immunizations; they also stick their hands in their mouths. Obviously, make sure those around your baby are not sick, and trust your instincts. Gently tell people no if you need to. Blame it on the advice in this book, your pediatrician, or whatever else you want if you need to, but protect your baby.

Maybe you've heard of cocooning. The concept of cocooning is that you choose a small group of people who are allowed to be a bit closer to your baby those first few weeks. These are the people that should definitely have an up-to-date Tdap vaccine, along with any others you deem necessary (like flu, COVID-19, etc.). Allowing your baby to be around this group gives you a bit of balance—you can share your baby and get a bit of a break, but you don't have to open up to everyone just yet.

4

Sleep (Please!)

*"Do what you need to do in the moment to survive.
Things will look better in the morning."*

—Me

Out of all the chapters, this is the one that I would have read a dozen times over when I was a new mom. The advice I write here is a conglomeration based on hard-won experience, uncountable websites desperately read between the hours of 11 p.m. and 6 a.m., several books (most notably *Cherish the First Six Weeks* by Helen Moon), an online sleep training course, and a hired sleep therapist.

My first child didn't sleep through the night until he was 12 months old. (He's still not a great sleeper at nearly five years old; in fact, I'm writing this chapter as I sit in the dark in his room, waiting for him to fall asleep.) With my second child, we knew what to do, or more specifically, what *not* to do, and the first time she slept through the night was at two months old (it took several more months to consistently do it every night, but there was progress).

One of the key things to understand is that babies need to learn how to do pretty much everything. Yes, this includes sleep. Your gentle and calm guidance goes a long way. You really shouldn't sleep train until at least four months old (and some pediatricians says five months). Before then, babies are just not developmentally ready. However, there are things that you can do before then that will help. Feel free to hold them while they sleep but try to do it *after* they've already fallen asleep. Give your baby a chance to soothe themselves and fall asleep, but if your baby is crying (actually crying, not just making noises, particularly before four months old), please go to them and soothe them by shushing, holding, rocking, pacifying, changing, or nursing them. It won't "spoil" them; it will just let them learn that you'll be there for them when they need you.

Night and Day Confusion

You may have heard that when your baby is born, they will have their nights and days confused. That's because your movement when doing things like walking around soothed them while they were in utero. Most likely, you moved most during the day and were still at night. The good news is that you can pretty quickly teach your baby when day and night really are once they are born.

Use the sun to help in this endeavor. Take walks and expose them to indirect sunlight in the mornings. Keep the lights on and the house at a normal volume during day naps. Talk to your baby and hold them. Make your nights the opposites of your days. Don't talk or interact with your baby during night feedings. Keep your room dark (I use a lamp with an orange light bulb so that I can see, but it's not too stimulating). Invest in blackout curtains and blackout film (it peels off; I have it on half of the windows in the nursery).

Awake Times, Sleep Windows, and Sleep Cycles

It's useful to know how long to expect your baby to be awake. The first few days, the baby is very sleepy. Then, from about two to six weeks, they still sleep a lot but begin to get into a predictable pattern. They will be most alert the first time they wake up to begin the day. After they wake up from their first nap, they'll likely still be tired and simply want to eat and go back to sleep. After their second nap, they might be awake for a short period of time. Then, after their third nap and eating, they will likely be close to the "witching hour(s)." More on this in a bit, but they may have more trouble sleeping during this time, even though they're tired.

Newborns (birth to three months old) are sleepy a lot of the time, but that doesn't mean that their sleep is random. Generally, their awake times are 45 minutes to 90 minutes long (they get longer as the baby gets older). Start watching them for sleep cues (see next section) for warnings that they are tired and ready to sleep. It's easier to put down a tired baby than an overtired one.

This point takes me to sleep windows. There is a sort of golden time when a newborn will most easily go to sleep. This is around the 45-to-60-minute mark when they're very young and the 60-to-90-minute mark when they're a month or two old. You might think you don't need to help them go to sleep; when they're tired, you rationalize, they will sleep. This is unfortunately not always the case. Babies need our help to learn to sleep. This means when they exhibit sleep cues, you should stop interacting with them (or they can get overstimulated), swaddle them, and put them in their bassinet or crib (with white noise, pacifier, or patting, if needed).

Finally, babies have sleep cycles, just like we do. We all wake briefly throughout our sleep. Adults' sleep cycles are about 90 minutes (sometimes a bit longer), whereas babies' sleep cycles are about 45 minutes long (sometimes a bit shorter). At the end of a cycle, they are in light sleep and may wake up. The same goes for us adults, but we've learned to connect our sleep cycles, so we might not even notice that we wake up. As parents, we need to help teach our babies to connect their sleep cycles.

Connecting sleep cycles is easy in theory—if the baby's environment is the same as when they first fell asleep, they will have a much easier time not waking up fully and staying asleep for another sleep cycle (45 minutes or so). If their environment is different (for instance, if they fell asleep being held and bounced and wake up alone in a bassinet), they will have a harder time falling back asleep. They're going to want that movement and physical connection again to go back to sleep. Rocking or bouncing them is easy when they're tiny and seven pounds, but it becomes much harder when they're more alert after a month or two and weigh 12 to 15 pounds. Plus, you don't want to continuously be needed every 45 minutes throughout the night to help your baby sleep because this means *you* won't be getting a full sleep cycle, which will make you feel even more tired than you would otherwise. That is why keeping things consistent, especially for night sleep, is important. At night, keep the white noise on and the room dark and boring. Try to put your baby down calm but awake, or wake them up ever so slightly once they're in the crib. This way their environment is the same when they wake up as when they fell asleep, helping them to connect those sleep cycles and sleep more deeply.

Time to Sleep? Sleep Cues

Babies need help to do everything, but they do give you some clues sometimes. Babies will tell you when they're tired. Look for these cues when they are near the end of their wake window. Many of the cues have to do with the eyes: rubbing their eyes, red eyes, and staring off into the distance without focusing. Yawning is a very clear cue for sleep, but it can actually be a sign that they are overtired or overstimulated. Crying is definitely a sign that they are overtired and possibly overstimulated, and you should try to avoid letting it get to that stage.

Speaking of crying, you may eventually be able to distinguish between your baby's different cries. However, don't feel bad if you can't. I wasn't able to with my first. There are cries for hunger, fear, tiredness, anger, discomfort and pain. Checking off the possibilities lets you better distinguish what the cries mean and what your baby needs. For example, if you fed them recently, their diaper has been changed, they have been thoroughly burped, have recently pooped, are warm and dry, and they're not overstimulated, then there is a good chance they are tired.

Witching Hour(s)

One of the most frustrating parts of a baby's schedule is the witching hour. It's usually between the hours of 5 p.m. and 9 p.m.; it starts soon after birth and peaks around the sixth week of life. Basically, this time is when your otherwise pleasant baby simply cannot be easily calmed and is resistant to sleep, and it seems like all they want to do is nurse or drink their bottle.

This is a tough time as a parent, especially if you have other kids and are trying to manage dinner and bedtime. You may feel as if you are constantly holding, rocking, and shushing your baby. It's a great time to enlist the help of another adult and take turns, as well as babywear (putting your baby in a baby carrier strapped to your chest). This frustrating time eventually passes. Just remember your baby is human too, and they are allowed to be grumpy at the end of the day, just like you can be at times.

Don't mistake the witching hour for colic. This fussy time is very common for babies. One reason for their fussiness is that they are tired and overstimulated, so try to get them to sleep. Also, this period can coincide with the time of the day babies want to cluster feed—that is, eating more frequently than normal. If your baby is near a growth spurt (between two to three weeks old, six weeks old, and three months old), then go ahead and feed them an extra time or two. Otherwise, if they can be soothed by other methods, do that instead.

Sleeping through the Night and Sleep Training

"Sleeping through the night" is actually defined as six to eight hours, so don't expect your baby to sleep for 10 to 12 hours straight when they are still fairly young. You can help your baby get to this point gradually by going from three hours between feeds at night to three-and-a-half to four and longer. Doing this consistently will pay off. If your baby wakes during the night before it's time to feed, don't go to them if they're not crying. If they are, try to soothe them while they're in their crib by patting them, shushing them, or putting their pacifier back in. Even if you have to pick them up to soothe them, try not to feed them unless you've tried everything else. Note that "soothed" doesn't mean sleep necessarily; if they're not full-out crying, don't feed them. This will teach them to go longer stretches between feeds. Plus, if you keep it fairly boring (don't talk to them), they'll soon learn that night is boring and they should sleep.

The typical recommendation is to not begin sleep training until a baby is at least four or five months old. At this point, they should be big enough to sleep longer stretches at night. But you can help your baby learn to sleep better before they're four to five months old. Waiting until they're actually crying is an important part of teaching them to connect sleep cycles and sleep longer. If they're simply grunting or making similar noises, let them. If they cry out a time or two and then stop, don't go to them. They may very well go back to sleep. Try waiting 30 seconds or a minute after they start crying consistently before going to them (start your count over if they stop). Eventually, you will be able to go longer stretches if you decide to sleep train. It's harder on Mom, really. You're just giving your baby a chance to try to self-soothe.

Since this book primarily focuses on the newborn stage (zero to three months), I won't cover sleep training in depth. What I will say is that with my first baby, I didn't want to sleep train. I believed he would learn to sleep on his own. When it became apparent a few months in that this wouldn't happen, we began sleep training with the gentlest no-cry method. That transitioned into pick up, put down—just like it sounds: pick up to soothe, then put down and repeat as necessary. That transitioned into a graduated cry-it-out method: let them cry for five minutes at first, then 10, etc.

Finally, when he was 12 months old and nothing had worked, and I was getting up six to eight times overnight in a 12-hour period to nurse or hold him, we did the full cry-it-out Ferber method. It worked in two days. With my daughter, we used the Ferber method at four months old—she was already a much better sleeper because I was experienced and not making the same mistakes as with my first. It worked after just one night. Was it unbelievably hard to hear my baby cry for an hour or two while we sleep trained them? Yes. Was it worth it to not have sleepless nights for months? In my eyes, yes. You may not want to sleep train or may choose a different option, but you're not a bad parent if you need to do so, even if they cry a lot those first few nights. Some babies just respond to different techniques.

What about formula-fed babies? Will they sleep through the night sooner? This is a myth I hear a lot, especially from older generations. All of the peer-reviewed research I have read simply doesn't support it though. Whether they're breastfed or fed with bottle and formula, if your baby isn't sleeping through the night, they're either legitimately hungry or there's something else going on.

Safe Sleep Guidelines

The American Academy of Pediatrics updated their safe sleep guidelines in 2022.[1] You can read a summary on their website or the full research paper, and you can talk to your pediatrician if you have questions. In short, the guidelines are:

- Put your baby on their back to sleep every time they sleep (including naps), using a firm, flat, noninclined sleep surface, for the first year.
- Feed your baby breast milk (if possible).
- Have your infant sleep in the parents' room but on a separate surface designed for infants, ideally for at least the first six months.
- Keep soft objects (e.g., pillows, blankets, toys) away from your infant's sleep area.

---

1 Moon, Rachel Y., et al. "Evidence base for 2022 updated recommendations for a safe infant sleeping environment to reduce the risk of sleep-related infant deaths." *Pediatrics*150.1 (2022): e2022057991.

- Offer a pacifier at nap time and bedtime. If you're breastfeeding, wait to introduce a pacifier until breastfeeding is consistent and comfortable and you have a good supply and effective latch.
- Avoid smoke and nicotine exposure, and avoid alcohol, marijuana, opioids, and illicit drug use during pregnancy and after birth.
- Make sure your baby isn't overheated, and don't cover their heads while they're sleeping (e.g., with a hat).

There are several additional guidelines and explanations under each of those points. I don't follow them all perfectly. For example, none of my babies slept in our room for the first six months. It just didn't work for us. I would venture that the first recommendation—back to sleep— is the most important; it's very likely why they list it first. I'd recommend consulting with your pediatrician if you decide to deviate from the safe sleep guidelines.

Sample Newborn Schedule

With my first baby, I breastfed on demand. However, that quickly turned into nursing every time he cried. It meant I really didn't know what he actually needed; I just tried to solve everything with nursing. This works a lot of the time but is exhausting to you and inefficient for your baby. Instead, you can put your baby on a loose schedule pretty much from the time they come home from the hospital. Here's a sample schedule that has worked well for me. No, you don't need to stick to it perfectly, but it does help to know when you might expect your baby to be a bit more alert or sleepy. As for feeding, do it after they wake up (not right before they fall asleep). This timing is critical. It's very important for your baby to avoid associating the bottle or breast with sleep. It can be hard at first because babies are so relaxed when they're eating that they often fall asleep. If this happens, try to wake them up—even if it's just for a few minutes—so they fall asleep without that association. As they get older, you can stretch out this awake period to play with them.

Note: the first three to four weeks, your baby may eat more frequently during the day (every two and a half hours or so) and at night (every three hours or so). Remember, babies' tummies are small, so they need to eat frequently. They need to sleep frequently as well: 14 to 17 hours per day is a good rule of thumb.

A sample schedule for a six week old is below, which follows the important eat, play, sleep pattern.

Six-Week-Old Schedule

7:30 a.m.: Happy wake up and eat.

8:00 a.m. (or when finished eating): Play—this will likely be your baby's most alert time.

8:30 a.m.: Put down in their crib to sleep. Younger babies may go to sleep earlier, while older babies may go to sleep later.

10:30 a.m.: Wake up and eat. Younger babies will sleep right after, whereas older ones (two-months and older) may want to be awake for an hour or so.

1:30 p.m.: Wake up and eat. This time, after they're done, your baby might want to be awake and interact with you, or they might want to go right back to sleep. Follow your baby's lead, but don't let them be awake for longer than 60 to 90 minutes.

4:15 p.m.: Wake up and eat.

4:45 p.m.: Play for about an hour.

5:45 p.m.: Sleep until 6:30/6:45 p.m., then awake (interacting with the family, bath time, etc.) until 7 p.m.

7:00 p.m.: Eat and sleep for the night. Keep the room quiet and dark from this time on.

10:00 p.m.: Dream feed. Even if they are sleeping, wake them to eat. Really try to get a full feed because after this you will go to bed as well.

2:00 a.m. (or longer if they let you!): Eat and sleep. Keep interaction to a bare minimum. Change their diaper in between breasts or halfway through the bottle. Really try to make your baby go at least three hours between feeds at night. Enlist your significant other to hold them to sleep if necessary. Feeding should be a last resort if they haven't gone at least three hours between eating. They'll soon get used to waiting and sleep until it's time to eat.

5:00 a.m.: Eat and sleep. If they wake up less than three hours before their wake-up time, you might not want to give them a full feeding. This is so you make sure the wake-up feeding is a full one. If they wake up less than an hour before their scheduled wake-up time of 7:30 a.m., try to get them back to sleep without feeding.

7:30 a.m.: Wake up and repeat!

Again, this is just a sample schedule that has worked for me. If the baby wakes up early, I try to get them back to sleep, even if I need to hold them. You really don't want an overtired baby, trust me. Just like you could wake up early and be fine for a bit, so can they, but eventually it will catch up to them (and you).

You'll notice that the sample schedule has the first night feeding 4 hours after the dream feed. You may have to work up to this gradually, by 15-minute intervals if necessary. One day, you'll be able to drop down to just one night feed, and then drop night feeds all together. You'll get there!

You may feed your baby more often during the day. Oftentimes, I find myself going two and a half hours in between feeds during the day. That's fine if it works for you. I always think that it's better to sneak in another feeding during the day than to have them be hungry (and thus wake up more) at night. Eventually, you'll work up to every three hours during the day, and later you will stretch that even longer. Night feeds will become more infrequent as well when your baby gets older, eats more, and learns to connect their sleep cycles.

Soothing Tricks

Soothing tricks basically come down to tricking your newborn into thinking that they're back in the womb. They should be warm (though not hot, and don't use hats while sleeping) and fairly contained. Legs should be free to move for hip health, but those arms should have limited movement to stop the startle reflex from waking them. This can be accomplished with a swaddle. A limited number of parents claim their newborn didn't like being swaddled, and their "evidence" is that they would break out of the swaddle. Experts and many parents agree that you should absolutely swaddle until baby can roll over. You can't use a blanket at this age, so the swaddle keeps them warm, and importantly, they feel safe and it prevents the startle reflex. If your newborn breaks out of a swaddle, try a different kind. (See the next section for swaddle suggestions.)

On to other soothing techniques. You may have heard of the Five Ss. This term, coined by Dr. Harvey Karp, includes swaddle, side stomach position, shush, swing, and suck. We covered swaddle. Side stomach should be for soothing purposes only. Since 1994, the National Institute of Health has promoted a Back to Sleep campaign to help reduce sudden infant death syndrome (SIDS). Thus, the side stomach position is for soothing only, not sleeping. Once the baby is calmed and drowsy, put them on their back in their crib.

One of the most indispensable tips is shushing, or white noise. I almost always use it when the baby sleeps. Daycare doesn't allow this, which is one reason I think my babies sleep more poorly there. Your womb is a loud place, and white noise helps recreate that. There are also the lesser-known pink and brown noises, which are not quite as sharp-sounding as white noise. Any of these are fine for your baby. You can use apps on your phone (e.g., White Noise—well named), and there's even a way to get white noise on your phone without an app (at least on iPhones through the accessibility settings). There are also plenty of white noise machines, both portable and for home. I like the Hatch Rest for home and the Dreamegg for travel, but I'm sure others are great too.

How loud should the white noise be? I always struggle with this question. From what I've read, it should be okay to play it all night at about 60–65 decibels. I have found that the 45–50 range is sufficient if they're calm. You can download free apps on your phone to check the decibel level, or some smart watches (like the Apple Watch) have it built in. A good rule of thumb is if it's too loud or uncomfortable for you, it's too loud for the baby. It's important to make sure the machine isn't right next to the baby's head. You can certainly have it higher to soothe them, and indeed sometimes that might be the only thing that works if they're screaming! But once they've calmed down, turn the volume down to a safe level (gradually, or they'll notice).

Swinging helps calm them as well. My pediatrician said it uses their nervous system against them. I prefer to think that it uses their nervous system *for* us parents. It's why newborns love to be bounced up and down and swayed side to side. Think of the Pilates mantra—up an inch, down an inch—at a bit of a faster pace. Your calves and thighs will certainly get a workout.

As for sucking, I recently came across the term "nonnutritive sucking." That really clicked for me. Babies are soothed by sucking, but more than that, they *need* to suck. My first baby used my breasts as a pacifier. That sucked (pun intended). With my third baby, we started using a pacifier about two weeks in. He never experienced nipple confusion, and he's not reliant on it once it falls out if he's sleeping. If he is struggling to relax enough to fall sleep, we can put in a pacifier, he sucks it for a minute or so, and then he's out like a light. My favorite pacifier is the Tommee Tippee lightweight one for newborns. My baby keeps it in his mouth most easily (this makes a huge difference when you're in the car and you can't reach back to pop it back in or at night). I've also tried Philips Avent pacifiers and MAM. Both are fine but harder for him to hold in by himself.

An added bonus from the pacifier is that my son takes a bottle easily (I really hope I don't jinx myself by writing that). My daughter absolutely refused a bottle. We tried nearly a dozen kinds, with all manner of tricks (see chapter 5 on breastfeeding for more), yet she refused to take it for a long, long time. That was terrible when I had to go back to work, and she had to go to daycare. I'm hoping my younger son finds the transition smoother. If your baby struggles to hold their pacifier in, you can try the reverse psychology trick of slowly pulling it out just a little. Chances are they'll suck harder to keep it in. This also works with breastfeeding.

The key to a lot of these soothing tricks is preventing your baby from relying on them to go to sleep; otherwise, when they wake up 45 minutes later and the swinging and sucking is gone, they may wake up fully and need you again to fall back asleep. It's much easier said than done but try to put your baby in their safe sleep space calm but awake. You can even try waking them up slightly once they're in their crib or bassinet. Hopefully they wake up for a few seconds and fall back asleep. You may have to go through the motions of soothing them again if they wake up fully, but eventually, it will pay off. It's much easier to bounce a seven-pound baby than a 15-pound one.

If they fully wake up immediately when you put them down, or when you stop patting or doing other soothing techniques, you can try to do it gradually, including "the hover." This is when you take off your hand (say, from their chest) and simply hover an inch or so above where it was. It's strange, but it's almost like a baby can sense that phantom contact. Their eyes may flutter open, but hopefully, they will drift right back to sleep.

I've covered the main ways to soothe that are often suggested. Here are a few others that I've learned from being a mom:

Your baby might need a change of scenery. Going outside almost always does the trick for me. It doesn't necessarily make them sleep, but it calms them for at least a minute or so if they've been screaming. Standing while holding your baby can also help, if you're not already. Somehow the baby feels the change in your body position, even if everything else you're doing is the same. Wrapping them in a baby carrier is very soothing. You might have been holding them closely to your chest, but the baby carrier is magic, especially bouncing or walking around. Plus, your hands are free to do other things (like write this book, if you're me).

Firmly patting the baby's butt or back can help as well. I'll do this when my babies are swaddled in their cribs if they're waking up, and it oftentimes prevents me from having to pick them up. It helps out of the crib as well. I've also noticed that some of my babies like having their legs elevated (about six inches or so) when they're in their cribs. If this sounds like your baby, but they wake up when their legs are put down, try the rolled blanket trick. Roll a blanket so that it's about four to six inches tall and stuff it in their swaddles under their legs. The blanket won't be loose, and their legs will stay elevated.

If your baby likes being held upright, you could try this trick, emailed to me by the Happiest Baby customer service: place a one-pound bag of rice on the baby's chest vertically (wrap with a cloth and secure with a rubber band). It mimics being held. This tip made me a bit nervous for unmonitored sleep, but if you are able to put it inside their swaddle, that could be okay. You could also try a weighted swaddle, like Dreamland Baby or Nested Bean. I'd recommend checking with your pediatrician regarding these options.

When your baby is a little older, they will eventually get sick. When mine are sick, they oftentimes want to be held to sleep and held upright. They can breathe more easily in this position; adding a humidifier to the room can also help. That's tough on you though, especially when you need to sleep! Maybe you've thought about slightly elevating the half of their bassinet or crib on the side closer to their head. Just get your pediatrician's approval first. The American Academy of Pediatrics recommends not doing this because if your baby slides down, their breathing could become compromised. If your pediatrician is on board and your baby's sleep is supervised, then it could be worth a shot. Just remember, don't put anything in the crib with your baby; instead, elevate one half of the bassinet itself (just three to four inches). There are some bassinets that sell products specifically for this purpose. If not, you could always try a heavy book.

What about the car? My babies sometimes fell asleep in the car, but never consistently and not if they were already riled up. I'd suggest not wasting the gas (and definitely not driving while sleep-deprived; that can be as bad as driving drunk!).

Finally, and this is easier said than done, try to keep calm. Your baby picks up on your stress. If you are calm and believe it will work, whatever you are doing has a better chance of soothing your baby. Take a break if you need to and remember they (and you) will eventually sleep.

Swaddle Suggestions

I have tried nine different swaddles. Here they are rated from best to worst.

Love to Dream Swaddle Up. You just put your baby in and zip up. Their arms stay in an up position, which apparently mimics their womb position. The tummy part is pretty tight, which probably helps them feel contained. I like this one a lot. 5/5

Dreamland Dream Swaddle. The entire thing is weighted. It has Velcro arms inside, and then you zip the rest over your baby. This is the priciest swaddle on this list. I like this one too; my baby's naps markedly improved when I switched to this swaddle. 5/5

Miracle Blanket. It's not that easy to use but has an extra flap that you wrap around the baby's arms and then under them so they can't get out. You wrap the small flap first, and then the larger flap around and around to secure them. It's great for Houdini babies. 4/5

Nested Bean. It has a little weighted pouch on their chest to help mimic the pressure of being held. A zipper runs along the sides and bottom, and the top has two buttons on each sleeveless shoulder. I tried this with my second baby with high hopes, and it didn't really improve sleep. Now they make a version that contains the arms, which I'd give a 4/5.

Snoo's Sleepea swaddle. I mainly use the Snoo swaddle, but that is out of necessity because I use a Snoo bassinet. Velcro straps secure the baby's arms, and then you zip the rest of the fabric over them. It does keep their arms contained usually, but not always. Also, with my second baby using it, I've noticed the Velcro occasionally failing. 3/5

HALO SleepSack. This is sort of the backward Sleepea. You zip the baby into the (sleeveless) swaddle first, and then use Velcro wings to wrap around the baby snugly. All of my babies have easily popped a hand or two out of these, so they're not my favorite. That being said, you can easily leave one arm out when they're older so that they learn how to self-soothe. My kids use these at daycare since I originally registered for so many of them. 3/5

Baby Merlin's Magic Sleepsuit. It's not really a swaddle but more of a transitioning product. Some people swear by it, but I didn't love it. It's a heavy, stiff suit that looks similar to a snowsuit. I had one but only used it once or twice as the safety is questionable, and it seems quite hot. 2/5

SwaddleMe. It has Velcro wings that wrap around the baby, but not as much Velcro as some other brands. It doesn't keep a baby's arms secure and is just okay in my opinion. 2/5

aden + anais swaddle blankets. These are traditional swaddles, which means they are a large, square piece of fabric that you fold your baby into. Chances are the nurses at the hospital used a cotton traditional type of swaddle on your baby those first few days. This brand is extremely popular, and people love buying them. So much so that I got over 30 at my baby shower, despite only registering for six. They are multipurpose—throw one in the diaper bag for an on-the-go changing table or nursing cover—but you definitely don't need more than three to six. Given that the fabric is fairly gauzy, I've never been able to wrap this blanket tightly enough where the baby can't escape. 1/5 for swaddling purposes, 5/5 for versatility.

Once your baby is a bit older and able to find their hand or grab a pacifier to self-soothe, the sleeveless sleep sacks are nice.

Contact Napping

Sometimes your baby just wants to be held. I always try to put them in their crib to nap first, for the reasons listed above. However, that's not always possible. In those cases, I hold my baby. I think doing that occasionally is great for bonding purposes, but you really don't want to get into the habit where you always have to hold them to sleep. They'll become heavier, you won't have spare time to yourself, and most importantly, they will get used to it. Then, when it's nighttime and you want to sleep as well, they won't understand why you can't just hold them like you normally do.

If you want to hold your baby while they sleep, try to let them fall asleep on their own in their crib before picking them up. I also believe in being flexible though. So, if your baby needs to nap on you in order to sleep, and it doesn't become a habit, that's perfectly okay. Baby wearing can make this easier on you. My babies have wanted to be held more often to sleep when they are sick. Luckily, they go back to sleeping in their cribs afterward, though it can take a night or two to reset.

Mistakes of a First-Time Mom

Now I'll share some of the mistakes I made as a first-time mom that I think contributed to my firstborn being a terrible sleeper.

I kept the house as quiet as possible and dark for his day naps. I would transfer him to his bassinet as carefully as possible when he was totally asleep instead of when he was drowsy but awake.

I went to him immediately for every noise he made while he slept, quickly picked him up, and nursed him. I thought I was being an amazing mom by being so responsive. I was not. Instead, I was interrupting his sleep and teaching him to be a light sleeper and to snack instead of get a full meal. I fed him as soon as he woke up in the morning and often nursed him to sleep. One of the best pieces of advice I ever got was to separate feeding from sleeping on *both* sides of sleep. By this, I mean waiting at least five minutes after my baby woke up in the morning to feed him (the advice was 20 minutes, but I found that wasn't practical for newborns). Then, at night, this meant feeding him at least 10 minutes before putting him down in his crib, totally awake. This advice was given to me by a sleep therapist we hired when my first son was a year old and still not sleeping through the night, but I still practice the morning part with my newborn by waiting a minute or two to feed him. He lays in his crib happily while I sing and open the curtains.

I've mentioned it a few times before, but babies are loud sleepers—leave them alone unless they are actually crying! Let them try to settle themselves down and wait a bit (count to 10 at a minimum or wait a minute if you can) before going to them. This will pay off in the long run as you won't be frequently waking your baby up accidentally. Also, be sure they are actually awake before going to them and trying to soothe them. Babies sometimes sleep with their eyes partially open. It's pretty impressive.

While I label some of the above behaviors as mistakes, teaching your baby to sleep is hard. I've been under pressure before: When I was pregnant with my first son, I was finishing my PhD and working full time. Teaching my kids to sleep (and motherhood in general) was much harder than that. Do what you need to do to survive in the moment. Make a plan before it's nighttime because good plans usually do not strike you at 4:30 a.m. after you've gotten roughly 90 minutes of fragmented sleep. You will have times when you doubt what you are doing and don't have any idea what to do. Your only job at that moment is to keep yourself and your child safe. It can help a bit to accept that you're going to be awake for the next hour (or more). That small mental shift can really make a difference. Take turns if you have another adult in the house. Things will look better in the morning, and you can make a better plan then.

5

Breastfeeding

"Don't cry over spilled milk. Unless it's breast milk.
In which case, cry a lot."

—Unknown

*B*reastfeeding is the most natural way to feed your baby. It's also the most convenient. That doesn't mean that it is easy or right for you. If you need or want to supplement with formula or not breastfeed at all, those are very valid options. Making sure your baby is fed is the best choice.

I breastfed all of my children. I also supplemented with formula after the first three months. This chapter is based on those experiences. Your journey may be different, and that's perfectly beautiful too.

Breastfeeding Benefits

First, the positives! Breastfeeding is really the most intimate experience shared between just you and your baby. The emotions that flood you (thanks to the oxytocin hormone) are a mix of a burst of joy and overwhelming love. I love all of my kiddos, of course, but when I nurse them and look at their tiny faces, nothing much comes close to that.

Breastfeeding is also super convenient and fast—no need to remember formula, water, bottles, or cleaning and sterilizing parts. You also don't need to worry about how to warm the bottle up when you're running errands or doing it quickly in the middle of the night. Importantly, you also don't have to worry (as much) about formula recalls or shortages. You just feed your baby.

It's rewarding to know you are providing your baby's sustenance physically and that it's the best they can get. Again, being fed is truly best, but breast milk does offer several advantages that formula cannot. Breast milk adapts to your baby's needs: it changes as they get older and when they get sick. For example, the first two to four days of life, your baby just gets tiny bits of colostrum—nutrient-, antibody-, and antioxidant-rich breast milk that is easy to digest and filling for your newborn's tummy. It then changes to thinner breast milk. Even within one feeding, the milk changes. At the beginning of a feed, the baby gets more foremilk, which is thinner and helps assuage their thirst. At the end of a feeding, they get more hindmilk, which is fattier and helps keep them full (and helps them pack on the pounds). It's technically all the same milk; it differs because the watery part of the milk moves down the ducts toward your nipple between feeds and thus comes out first.

There are additional great benefits for your baby's health. When they (or you) are sick, the antibodies in breast milk can help. Plus, there's research showing that white blood cells in breast milk significantly increase when you or your baby are sick. Furthermore, you might be glad to know that when you get a vaccine, those antibodies also pass along to your baby through your breast milk. This is helpful, especially when a baby is too young to receive the vaccine directly. For example, both of my older kids were under six months old during flu season and thus unable to get the flu shot. Luckily, I did get the flu shot and was breastfeeding them, so they got some level of protection. Breastfeeding has also been associated with a lower risk of sudden infant death syndrome (SIDS).

Of course, the benefits of passing things from your body to your baby through your breast milk also mean you should be careful about what you consume (like alcohol or caffeine). You can indulge, but practice moderation and time it so that there are at least two hours before you need to nurse again. And at the risk of sounding like a middle school campaign, definitely don't do drugs, for multiple reasons.

Finally, breastfeeding benefits you. It can help you bond with your baby because it increases oxytocin. It can also decrease your risk of some cancers, including breast cancer. Some really interesting studies have found that mothers who only nursed on one side had a much lower risk of cancer in that breast. See the CDC webpage for further benefits to Mom and babies.[2]

What Is Breastfeeding Actually Like?

When I was pregnant with my first son, I was nervous about breast-feeding. Having a little baby suck on my nipples for hours a day did not sound appealing. I wanted to try it because of all of the benefits, but I wasn't sure it would be the right thing for me.

Once my baby latched on the first time, I was surprised by how *natural* it felt. When they have a good latch, it doesn't feel like your nipple is constantly stimulated. It feels a bit like a tug or almost nothing at all. It's totally different from any sexual stimulation you may have experienced before, so don't worry about that. As a side note, I think this is why many women don't want their breasts touched sexually while they are frequently breastfeeding; it's nature's way of ensuring breasts are reserved for the baby when they're very young. We likely evolved with this aversion (along with a lowered libido) in order to discourage sex, and another potential pregnancy, until the current newborn was older.

A few seconds to a minute after your baby latches on, you may feel your breasts (one or both of them) get heavier or have a sense of pressure. This is called a let-down, and it can happen more than once during a feeding session. Until this happens, your baby usually sucks more shallowly and more quickly. Afterward, they slow down a bit with

---

2   "Breastfeeding: Recommendations and Benefits," Centers for Disease Control and Prevention, accessed March 12, 2024, https://www.cdc.gov/nutrition/InfantandToddlerNutrition/breastfeeding/recommendations-benefits.html.

a suck-suck-suck-long pull pattern. This is the baby gathering milk with a few sucks before swallowing.

You may have several let-downs in a nursing session, and sometimes it may feel stronger than other times.

How to Get a Good Latch

Your baby will naturally root around searching for your nipple. You can help them get a good, deep latch by compressing your areola with one hand, tickling your baby's chin with your nipple, waiting for them to open their mouth, and then quickly pulling their head toward your breast with your other hand. They should have a wide seal around your nipple and some of your areola, and their chin should touch your breast. Position them so their head and spine are in line (their tummy facing your tummy), and support their head and back with your hand.

If it doesn't feel quite right, you can gently use a finger to break the seal on the side of your breast (don't try to pull out your nipple without doing this because that might hurt). You can support your breast with the same-side hand. I hold my breast while nursing so that it's not too heavy for the baby and to help their mouth stay properly aligned.

There are various feeding positions. Tummy to tummy has worked best for me, but there are others you can look up if you don't like this.

Start on one side, and when your baby slows down or stops (or it's been enough time), switch sides. Always offer both breasts, if you can, and then start on the side you ended on the last time. You can download a nursing app on your phone to help you remember which side you started on, and you can use a physical reminder (like a hair band on a wrist or a burp cloth) as an easy reminder as well.

Breastfeeding Setup

What's most important here is convenience and comfort. It's nice to have a nightstand next to where you will be feeding your baby most often. You can put your drink, a snack, a book, etc. on it to reach easily. It's also great to have extra burp cloths, diapers, and wipes nearby. I used to move to the changing table to change the baby during a nursing session. Now, I just use my bed (during the early weeks when the baby is sleeping in the same room) or my lap (once the baby has moved to the nursery and I'm sitting in a rocking chair).

I like to have an orange or red light on for night feeds. This way, the baby doesn't get a cue that it's morning time. These colors promote good sleep. I use a lamp with an orange light bulb, but if you buy a white noise machine, some of them have built-in lights with different color options.

I like to place a burp cloth on one side of the nursing pillow and a waterproof, reusable changing pad on the other side. This has saved me countless times when the baby has had pee leak out of their diaper or a blowout during a nursing session. Plus, it has the added benefit of showing you which breast the baby last fed from (if you switch the burp cloth and changing pad when you switch breasts). While you might have an app on your phone to record nursing sessions and sides, the visual cue is helpful in the middle of the night when the baby just wants to eat and is impatient.

Finally, posture while breastfeeding is important. You're going to be picking up, holding, and nursing your baby a lot, so you need to protect your back. Try not to hunch over when you're feeding your baby. Support the arm that is holding your breast; you can use a pillow if you don't have an armrest. Try stretching or enlist your partner for a massage when you can.

The First Week of Breastfeeding

The first two to four days after birth, your body will produce colostrum, that thick, yellowish milk that is perfect for a baby at this age. Then, your milk will come in—colostrum is breast milk too, so it's technically already "in." You'll know this happens because it might sound like your baby is taking bigger swallows and your breasts may feel heavier, fuller, or firmer.

Your breasts are going through a lot this week. Unfortunately, it can be painful or uncomfortable as your nipples and breasts adjust. For example, the first few seconds of each nursing session were very painful for me for about the first two weeks with each baby. Some nursing challenges go away, but if they don't or it's making you unhappy, you may want to speak to a lactation consultant or switch to pumping or formula. That can be an emotional and difficult choice, but it doesn't mean it's not the right choice for you and your baby.

One final thing: if you are only or primarily breastfeeding, your baby will need a vitamin D supplement every day because breast milk doesn't provide enough (formula does). They sell infant-specific vitamin D drops, and it's easy to administer them. You should start it as soon as you come home from the hospital.

How Often Will Baby Eat and for How Long?

A general rule of thumb for the first two weeks is that your baby will eat every two and a half to three hours. From that point on, you can try to stretch it to every three hours. Night eating will gradually stretch even further, though day eating will pretty much stay at the every-three-hours rate for the entire newborn phase. Nursing sessions are timed from beginning to beginning. In other words, if I started to feed the baby at 1 p.m., the next session would likely start around 4 p.m.

Some guidelines will say you should "feed on demand" if you're breastfeeding. I disagree. I think for a first-time mom, this guidance can be incredibly hard to interpret. I tried to follow this advice with my first baby, and I ended up feeding him every time he cried because I thought he was hungry and I was responding to that cue. I was wrong. Babies cry for all sorts of reasons, hunger being a pretty important one, but sleep is too. I'd respond to every cry with the breast, and my baby would often latch on but quickly fall asleep. (They may latch even when not hungry because of the rooting and sucking reflexes.)

Therefore, we got into a terrible pattern where I would nurse him every 90 minutes or so, and he began to *need* to feed that frequently because he wasn't getting a full meal in! In other words, he was snacking, and it was exhausting for me to basically be constantly on call, nursing him. Because of this, I tried to make sure not to feed babies two and three before the two-and-a-half-to-three-hour mark. I tried to respond to crying in other ways: Did they need to be changed? Were they cold? Too hot? Did they just want to be held? Did they want nonnutritive sucking (through a pacifier)? Did they want to sleep but weren't sure how? This last one was usually the culprit. Especially if they're overtired, babies will cry. This loose nursing schedule worked much better; I was happier, and my babies were too.

It's still hard though. Your baby's need to eat so frequently can wear on you, especially because it's every three hours, 24/7. I remember feeling like a cow, particularly with my first son. Breastfeeding is rewarding, but it's also physically and mentally draining. The three-hour frequency doesn't take into account cluster feedings, when the baby wants to nurse more often. Cluster feeding often occurs during growth spurts: around two to three weeks, six weeks, and three months. It should only last a few days, though, so don't despair! You'll know it's cluster feeding because your baby won't be soothed by anything but eating. When they want to cluster feed, you'll need to break the every two and a half to three hours guideline and feed them more often. If you want, offer them a bottle instead to give your breasts a break.

In terms of duration, every mom will be different based on their milk supply, let-down speed, and how efficient the baby is. In my experience, during the first three weeks or so, a baby will nurse 15 minutes per side. You'll want to burp before offering the second breast and always offer both breasts. The next session, you'll start with the one you offered last. This way, each breast has a chance to be drained, which will stimulate your supply and prevent one breast from becoming engorged. My pediatrician told me more than 15 minutes per side is too long because the trade-off between the calories the baby gets versus expends nursing reaches a point of diminishing returns. With all the nursing, holding, burping, and diaper changing, a nursing session the first few weeks might take 45 to 60 minutes. That's especially hard in the middle of the night, so enlist your partner to help. They can also take the baby during the day so you can nap.

Your baby soon gets more efficient at nursing, which means the time they nurse per side will decrease. Around eight weeks old, my baby was at about 8 to 10 minutes per side, usually less on the second breast. This means a nursing session went down to about 25 to 30 minutes, including holding, diaper changing, and burping. I'll go over how to make sure a baby is getting enough milk in the next section, but if they seem content and your breasts are soft (not heavy or hard) after a session, those are good signs.

I mentioned you want to burp your baby. This is true of breastfed babies as well, although their burps may not always be as loud, and they may not burp as frequently as a bottle-fed baby (who takes in more air because the seal between their mouth and the nipple isn't as tight). You burp a baby to release the gas they may otherwise struggle to expel, and yes, you want to burp them even if they are peacefully asleep after nursing. You don't want to put them down to sleep only to have to get them 30 minutes later because they burped and spit up all over themselves. Burp them in between breasts and at the end of a session, or if they're pulling off from the breast a lot (they might be doing this because have built-up gas, which is uncomfortable).

So, how do you burb a baby? You can put them over your shoulder (high up on their torso to put pressure around their chest or belly) and pat them firmly. I also like sitting them on my leg, one of my hands under their chin to hold their head and the other patting firmly. If pats don't work, try gently lowering the baby onto their back and then raising them back up. That could dislodge the gas bubble. Rubbing firm circles up their back has also worked really well for me. If they haven't burped after a few minutes, you can move onto the other side or, if they're finished, hold them upright for 5 to 10 minutes to help them digest the milk. Then, put them down to sleep.

You might be wondering when night feeds will get spaced apart farther. Every baby is different, but I've found my second and third babies were able to go about four hours around one month, and my 10-week-old has had several nights going five or even six hours in between night feeds. The second night feed might come two and a half or three hours after that though. It really just depends on the night. I aim for progress overall and try to look week by week rather than day by day. Everyone will have an off day or two. Just try to get back on track and help your baby stretch out those night feeds by doing what you need to do to help them go to sleep. The hope is that it pays off soon and your baby learns to sleep until it's feeding time.

Is the Baby Getting Enough?

You want to make sure your baby is getting a nice, full feeding at each nursing session, for multiple reasons. As I've mentioned before, you want to avoid snacking (eating for five minutes or less). You also want to make sure they are healthy and gaining weight. So, how do you ensure these full feeds?

First, try to wait at least three hours between nursing sessions (from start to start). This way the baby is hungry and their belly is empty, ready to be filled. If they fall asleep at the breast before they're done, wake them up. Falling asleep is common, particularly at earlier ages, because the baby is so relaxed and has oxytocin in their brain (just like you!). To wake up your baby, walk your fingers up their back, undress them, change their diaper, blow on their face, burp them, or tickle their feet. I've found sniffing loudly or clearing my throat sometimes triggers the startle reflex and briefly wakes them. If all else fails, try rubbing a wet wipe or washcloth on their body (but don't let them get too cold). Try hard to wake your baby up to get a full feed in. You can also try pulling your nipple out slowly—they often suck it back in quickly and may eat for a little longer too.

If you are getting good, full feeds in, chances are your baby will be gaining weight. A rule of thumb is for a baby to gain one ounce per day, though you're probably not weighing them at home unless your pediatrician has recommended it. You'll be able to see their weight gain during your multiple pediatrician visits that first month.

Another good way to tell that your baby is getting enough food is that your breasts will be soft after a feed. Before a nursing session, your breasts will likely be heavier and larger, and you'll have a feeling of fullness or even a let-down as nursing time approaches. An additional telltale sign is that your baby will seem content once they finish eating. Finally, you can count their wet and dirty diapers to reassure yourself that your baby is having sufficient output (and thus input). While it can be tough to know whether or not a baby is eating sufficiently—especially when you're not bottle-feeding and can't see how many ounces they are eating—try to relax. If your baby seems happy, chances are they are getting enough food.

Try not to let your baby use you as a pacifier though. You'll notice they're doing this if they're chewing or gnawing more than sucking and swallowing, or if they're trying to nurse more often than they should and quickly fall asleep at the breast. Cluster feeding does not apply here, because they will actually be eating, not just chewing for comfort.

When Will the Baby Wean?

The American Academy of Pediatrics and the World Health Organization recommend breastfeeding until 24 months (or beyond). Both also recommend exclusively nursing until six months old. But in terms of weaning a baby, I don't think that there really is a right answer. It's up to you and your baby. My first weaned off naturally at 25 months. By the last month, he was only nursing once in the mornings. My second weaned off by herself at 13 months. Because they both did it at their own pace, I never got engorged and never had to do anything to help myself dry up. (Though I've heard that cabbage leaves work wonders if you need to do so.)

Just remember, if a baby weans prior to 12 months old, they will need to drink formula. If they wean after the first year, they can go straight to whole milk.

Breastfeeding Challenges and Issues

Breastfeeding is an incredible bonding experience and can be joyous, but it's also quite tough. Your freedom is limited—if you're exclusively breastfeeding, you're the baby's only source of nutrition those first few weeks or months.

Additionally, it can be hard to get started nursing. The baby may not latch well or stay latched; this lasts for a few days, though it improves quickly, in my experience. It can also be painful as your nipples get used to the near constant sucking. Your nipples can crack or develop milk blebs (a clogged pore that looks like a white spot on your nipple and can be painful). You might also have plugged milk ducts (research suggests the ducts are narrowed due to inflammation). I've had some of these symptoms, and what helped was nipple cream (lanolin-based), air drying my nipples after rubbing a bit of breast milk on them (it has healing properties), and heat. Some recommendations used to include vibration and massage, but updated research suggests *avoiding* massage, avoiding nipple shields, using ice if that provides symptomatic relief, and feeding on demand instead of until the breast is "empty." These symptoms go away after a week or two if you treat them.

You might also have engorged breasts (extra heavy or painfully hard breasts) that develop because you have an oversupply, the baby skips a feeding, etc. This can happen anytime throughout your breast-feeding journey. For me, it's more common when the baby is sick and not eating as frequently or at the end of a workday (because pumping was inefficient for me). If your breasts are engorged, pumping or nursing can help. This is when you would want to start on the engorged side when breastfeeding, even if you offered that same side first during the last feed. If you go the pumping route, remember that your body will think it needs to keep producing that much milk, so the problem will continue if your baby doesn't actually need that much. Instead, pump just enough to help with the pain and slowly reduce the time you're pumping. Heat can also help, like a warm bath or a warm, wet hand towel on your breasts. Engorgement goes away as soon as you empty your breasts sufficiently.

A nonpainful but embarrassing breastfeeding challenge is leaking. Your breasts may leak some breast milk that can go through your clothes if it's close to or past feeding time, or if you hear your baby crying. It can also happen to one breast when your baby is latched onto the other. You can put nursing pads in your bra to prevent breast milk from seeping through your clothes, or if you find it happening often, particularly during a nursing session, you can use a breast milk catcher (like the Elvie Catch) to save the milk.

Another common symptom is discomfort when you have your let-down, like there's too much pressure in your breasts. Luckily, this symptom usually resolves after a few seconds of your baby nursing. An additional not-so-fun side effect of breastfeeding: you stink! Yes, you may suddenly develop more potent BO. There's actually a reason behind this though, and that is, like many other things, thanks to evolution. Your stinky armpits help guide your baby to your breast and associate it with your unique (though smelly) smell. I only noticed this symptom with my third baby, and it went away after about five months.

Some more serious challenges of breastfeeding include thrush (itching, burning, flaking skin, or shooting pain; the solution is prescription medication), a stabbing or burning pain after nursing, and mastitis (fever and chills along with painful or burning breasts, usually treated with antibiotics). Luckily, I have not had these symptoms, but if you do, make sure to reach out to your doctor right away. They may want you to come in or may prescribe medication.

Finally, your baby may not be able to breastfeed well. For example, if they have a tongue tie, it may be harder for them to breastfeed. A tongue tie means they have a little flap of skin under their tongue attached to the bottom of their mouths. It restricts their range of motion but can be easily fixed with a simple surgery. It's also possible, though unlikely, that you develop sudden and intense negative emotions just before your let-down. This is called dysphoric milk ejection reflex, or D-MER, and while it's very short term, it can be concerning to you.

If you're experiencing any breastfeeding difficulties, talk to your doctor, your baby's pediatrician, and a lactation consultant. Sometimes, they can help you work through the problems, and you can still breastfeed. Other times, you may want or need to switch to pumping or formula, and that's great too.

Breastfeeding in Public

Breastfeeding in public is legally protected in every state, though some states do qualify this with something like "with as much discretion as possible." I've never had anyone say anything negative to me while I'm breastfeeding my child in public. In fact, the handful of people who have commented have usually said something like, "It's so wonderful that you're doing that."

That being said, it can be awkward to nurse in public. I use a nursing cover, though it's a personal comfort thing for me (it's not required). You may want to practice using a nursing cover a few times at home before doing it in public. It can be a little tough to see your baby with a cover on and help them latch. The cover may also fall onto their face, which makes it uncomfortable for them. I try to hook the cover over my bent knee to prevent this, though it sometimes falls back.

To position the baby, I usually use the cradle or cross-cradle holds. I have a long torso, so I like to prop up my knee closer to the baby's head by putting that side's foot on my other knee. This elevates the baby a little and is convenient when you don't have a nursing pillow. You don't have to wear a nursing top to breastfeed in public. If you don't and you have to lift up your shirt to access your breasts, you might want to wear a tank top underneath so your midriff isn't exposed.

Pumping

Pumping has always been incredibly inefficient for me, and when I have had my last pumping sessions, I've celebrated. I'm a working mom, and my kids go to daycare. I knew I was going to have to pump if I wanted to continue breastfeeding (which I did). I started out with the Spectra S1 pump, which was fine. It was fairly quiet and compact, but I wasn't producing as much as I had hoped. At most I'd get three ounces or so per session (throughout my entire pumping path), and near the end of my pumping (around 10 months old), the babies would be taking six to eight ounces of milk per feeding. Therefore, I simply wasn't pumping enough.

I tried to increase my milk supply with lactation teas, various lactation bars (BOOBIE* Bars are delicious), and lactation supplement pills. I also tried a hospital-grade pump (which you can rent). I knew my supply at home was fine because my baby seemed satisfied after nursing sessions in the morning, at night, and on the weekends. I was also quite full at the end of a workday. Pumping just didn't work well for me; my body knew the pump wasn't my baby. So, I supplemented with formula for daycare days.

How does pumping actually work, and what can help smooth the process? Traditional pumps use flanges and air to mimic a baby suckling at the breast. Good pumps will allow you to alter the speed and intensity of the sucking, and many have different modes to encourage a let-down (using faster sucking) and then stronger, slower sucking after.

Some pumps will even switch for you automatically as they detect the amount of milk coming out.

The Elvie Pump will do this. I got this pump with my first baby back when it was only being sold in the UK (when it was first released). I had to do some tricky post office shuffling, but I got it sent to my address in the US. Now, the Elvie Pump is widely available. It's a great pump; it's very tiny (can fit in your nursing bra), it's free of tubes and wires (traditional pumps have long tubes that connect the flanges to the pump), and it's very quiet, though it's not silent. It also makes your boobs look artificially huge, so I wouldn't pump while running errands and definitely not at work while interacting with colleagues. But I do still highly recommend it. The Elvie connects to an app so you can see how much you're pumping in real time. It also has automatic switching between different modes so you can take advantage of multiple let-downs.

Regardless of what pump you choose, one thing that will really help with the amount you pump is ensuring a proper flange fit. Women's nipple sizes differ. You can get a nipple ruler to help you determine the correct size; these rulers have holes of various sizes that you put your nipple in to measure the fit (yes, really). The correct size helps make sure your nipple won't be too sore after pumping and that you maximize the amount of milk you're getting. You can also get flange inserts to aid with fit and comfort.

In addition to those things, when you actually pump, here are some suggestions that can help: smelling a shirt or other clothing your baby has worn, manually compressing your breasts, putting warming pads on your breasts (heat helps with let-down), doing the same things you do while nursing (like watching a TV show or reading), and importantly, relaxing while you're pumping. This last one is easier said than done, particularly if you're stressing about your output. If you're stressed, it becomes a vicious cycle. Remember, you are doing the best you can for your baby, and you can always use formula if you need or want to.

Just like with bottles, you'll need to clean your pump parts. It's useful to have multiple sets so you don't have to wash them after every pump. When I pump at work, I put my pump parts in a wet-dry bag in the refrigerator in between pumping sessions. That way I don't have to wash them until the end of the day.

To store your breast milk, you can pour your pumped milk directly into a bottle (some pumps let you pump directly into a bottle), or you can use breast milk storage bags. I like the ones by Lansinoh and Medela that you can stand up or lay down flat to freeze, saving you storage space. As a side note, if you've ever wondered about the expression "don't cry over spilled milk," know that it is perfectly acceptable to cry over spilled breast milk. I once spilled four ounces of just-pumped milk and had a mini breakdown in my work's pumping room.

Finally, if you don't have a pump on hand, you can use hand expression or a manual pump. As you might imagine, this isn't as efficient as an electric pump or a baby. But it can help with engorgement in a pinch. You can also do it in the shower. The water, warmth, and relaxation can be helpful. The Haakaa is a popular manual pump that you compress and place on your breast, and the pressure can pull out the milk. You can also use something like the Elvie Catch, which goes in your bra and simply catches the milk that can be released when your baby is nursing at the other breast.

Formula

Formula is a great choice if you decide you don't want to breastfeed, you try and find out that you can't (or no longer want to), or you want to supplement. While the decision to use formula was very emotionally frustrating for me with my first baby, by the second, I had accepted that my body didn't respond well to pumping and that I would breastfeed when I was with my baby and give them formula when they were at daycare or with a sitter. (I still pumped to maintain supply and reduce engorgement.) I gave myself more grace and let go (mostly) of the mom guilt.

There are many different types of formula. You should try to get one that has sufficient DHA. Some are organic, while others aren't. All of the ones I have seen have enough vitamin D, but you should make sure yours does.

Enfamil, Gerber, and Similac are the major brands of formula. Many have formulas for sensitive stomachs. With my first baby, I used Enfamil NeuroPro and then Enfamil Gentlease when he had tummy troubles. With my second baby, I did a formula taste test of seven different kinds. I was shocked at how terrible most of them tasted (I've tried my breast milk, and it is decidedly better tasting, if I do say so myself—like sweet milk). I thought Similac tasted better than Enfamil, but neither tasted good. I ended up going with Earth's Best Organic because it tasted the most similar to breast milk. I also like Happy Baby Organic formula. Buy what works for you and your baby.

Bottles

The first few months, while I was on maternity leave, I breastfed my first two babies exclusively. This backfired with my second baby because she avidly refused to take a bottle when I sent her to daycare, which was very problematic. We tried giving her a bottle at about two months old to get her used to it, and nothing worked. I tried 10 different types of bottles, different formulas, breast milk in a bottle, different people feeding her, different methods of feeding her, temperatures, you name it. Being fed by others, using a bottle with a latex nipple, and running the nipple under warm water seemed to help a bit, but ultimately, she kept refusing no matter what.

Once she started daycare, she relented after about a week of starving herself throughout the day. That was really tough, and with my third baby, we introduced a bottle once a week starting when he was about four weeks old. He took to it much better and never had nipple confusion. He also takes a pacifier, which my daughter did not. This may have also helped with taking the bottle. Overall, I definitely recommend introducing a bottle sooner rather than later. You can pump so that your supply doesn't go down if you don't want to use a bottle every day at the same time.

There is an unbelievable number of bottle brands out there, all claiming to be the best and most like the breast. Really, what I've found is that your baby will likely get used to whatever you consistently give them. My first used Philips Avent and Comotomo, and my second and third babies use Lansinoh. I like the feel of Lansinoh most, but pulling the nipple through the screw cap is easier (doesn't pop through) on the Philips Avent.

You need to clean your bottles well. Most brands have you boil the parts for about five minutes before using them for the first time. Then, you can wash them with hot water and dish soap. Many brands are also dishwasher-safe, though I don't like doing that for the nipples because it seems to wear them out more quickly. For these, I find it's best to use a bottle brush that has a nipple attachment in order to get them thoroughly cleaned. After they are washed, you can sterilize the parts in a bottle sterilizer if you want. I do this when the baby is a newborn (i.e., the first three months) but then stop after that. I try to rinse the bottles with water as soon as the baby's done eating so nothing really gets stuck to form bacteria.

Infant Diet after Milk

Here's a quick section on when and what your baby will eat when they're ready for solid food. My pediatrician recommended starting solids at the four-month mark. This was earlier than I anticipated (I had always read that solids would start at the six-month mark). However, once you start solids, it takes a long time for the baby to get the hang of it. My babies weren't eating solids in any significant way until at least six months old. It took them that long to not choke on the thicker-than-milk (though still very thin) food and not have it dribble out of their mouths.

My pediatrician recommended giving the baby oatmeal cereal first and then meats. Yours may be different. You can also thin out pureed solids with breast milk or formula, if they're too thick. Try and try again; your baby will probably act like they don't like it at first. You're supposed to introduce a food and then wait a few days to see if the baby has a reaction. We did this with my first, but with my second, we really didn't. Introduce all manner of foods that first year, including allergens. We buy a baby oatmeal by Ready. Set. Food! that includes various allergens (e.g., milk, egg, peanut, soy).

One thing you shouldn't give a baby before 12 months old is honey because it may have bacteria that can cause infant botulism. This illness can cause your baby to have muscle weakness, a weak cry, and difficulty breathing. It's incredibly rare, but very serious, so avoid honey. You should also stay away from undercooked and unpasteurized foods for their safety. Give them only formula or breast milk when they're under 12 months old (no cow's milk). Avoid water when your baby is younger than six months old, and even after that, prioritize formula or breast milk. Ask your pediatrician about your infant's diet if you have questions.

6

Postpartum Care

"Taking care of you matters too. Period."
—Me

You've just had a baby! Now you, your family, and your friends are squarely focused on that infant. But what about *you*, separate from your baby? Even though you're right to focus on your baby, prioritize yourself as well. You've heard the airplane announcement: put your own oxygen mask on before you help your child. Something similar is applicable here. If you don't take care of yourself, you won't be able to effectively take care of your baby.

First Bowel Movement and Peeing

I've read that some moms fear pooping for the first time after labor even more than labor itself. Yes, it's a bit scary, especially if you've gotten stitches. The best things you can do for yourself are to drink plenty of water and take the stool softener your nurse will give you at the hospital. Also, don't try to avoid it; that will only make things worse. Just breathe, try not to strain, and let go. It'll be okay.

Peeing can sting a bit, and it's why your nurse will give you a peri bottle. You fill it with warm water and squeeze that onto your urethra while peeing. This helps to alleviate the sting. You can take home the peri bottle from the hospital. I like to have one in each bathroom of the house; you'll be using it frequently for at least a week. One more thing—pat, don't wipe. This will help avoid aggravating your swollen and irritated skin.

First Shower

You'll shower in the hospital, which will feel fantastic. The hospital towels are scratchy, thin, and tiny, but you'll also be bleeding, so I'd use them instead of bringing your own towel if I were you (also bring your own shampoo and conditioner). Be gentle when lathering up, don't use soap on your vulva (the outside part), and don't even think about using soap in your vagina (the inside part). If you're breastfeeding, also don't use soap on your nipples. It can wash off the natural lubricant and change the smell for your baby.

As a side note, this advice isn't just for the first few days after giving birth. You're not really supposed to use soap on your vulva and definitely not in your vagina. I learned this from my OB-GYN when I was 27 years old. No one had ever told me this before. The only reason she said anything is because I was a few weeks postpartum and mentioned a burning feeling on my vulva when I was showering. Apparently, it was because I was using soap. I can't stand the thought of not using soap down there, so now I use a pH-balanced, unscented soap (the brand I use is called Tree to Tub). It's expensive, but I only use it for my vulva, so it lasts a while.

Lochia and Vagina Care

Remember how during those nine months of pregnancy you didn't have a period? It's one of the few nice things about pregnancy, in my opinion. Well, the joke's on you because after labor, all that blood you've avoided will come at you at full force.

Lochia is the vaginal discharge you'll experience for the next four to eight weeks after birth that contains blood, mucus, and uterine tissue (not the prettiest definition). It gradually tapers off, and mine went away completely by about six weeks. But this is one reason why you shouldn't go swimming for those first few weeks after birth (no tampons for you!). Use those huge overnight, extra-long pads to soak up the blood. I also suggest getting some postpartum underwear (like Frida Mom) that you can simply throw away. You'll only need these for about the first week.

Frida Mom also has an ice pack and pad combination, which can be nice when you're at the hospital (the hospital ice packs often leak). However, you really won't need ice packs after you get home from the hospital (at least I did not). Witch hazel pads or spray are nice to have to aid with stinging. To use them, put a period pad in your underwear and then witch hazel pads along the length of it (or spray). Call your doctor if you soak through more than one pad per hour, if you pass a clot bigger than a golf ball, or if you experience flu-like symptoms.

As for your regular period, many women start having theirs again sometime between six and 12 weeks after delivery. I mainly breastfed my kids, and I started my period 13 months after birth with each of them. There's a wide range of "normal."

To regain strength, you can do Kegels (a pelvic floor muscle exercise) right after birth. If you haven't done these before, you use the muscles that start and stop the flow of urine. Start off with a few and build up speed, repetitions, and hold time. This will help with a wide range of things, including supporting your internal organs, avoiding incontinence, and making sex more pleasurable. If you're experiencing pain or incontinence, tell your doctor. They may refer you to a pelvic floor physical therapist.

Diet

The good news here is that you can eat everything again. Yes, that includes alcohol, even if you're breastfeeding. You just have to time it properly and practice moderation. The best time to indulge is right after a nursing session. Ideally, you want two hours between the time you finish your drink and the time you have to nurse again. That way the alcohol is out of your system (and out of your milk). Moderation means limiting it to one drink. Given that you've been sober for at least nine months, this should be plenty (I was definitely feeling my first half glass of wine postpartum).

I also like to practice this timing and moderation rule when it comes to caffeine and medicine. This way, I limit what is passed onto the baby as much as possible. It shouldn't affect them much, but I have read that breastfed babies whose mothers drink lots of caffeine can become jittery and hard to put to bed. You definitely don't want that because then you will likely need more caffeine!

Your (Changed) Body

You went through a lot, both physically and emotionally, during pregnancy and labor. Most women I know don't "bounce back." The reality is that you will most likely never again look exactly how you did before becoming pregnant. And that's okay.

It took nine, nearly 10, months to grow a baby. Give yourself at least that much time to lose the weight you gained. You might have to come to terms with the fact that you may never lose it all. Most people will understand, although men are notoriously obtuse about this (my husband has been great, but certain other adult males have commented in ignorance). My four-year-old loves to say, "Mommy, is there a baby in your tummy?" I'm eight weeks postpartum, and he just likes to say it because he knows it annoys me, much like he likes to say, "Mommy, you *love* chocolate, right?" (I do not.)

Your body is telling the story of how you carried new life into this world and survived labor. That's worth celebrating. So, what has potentially changed? You may have stretch marks (despite all the creams out there, it mostly comes down to genetics), and you may be curvier. If you're breastfeeding, your breasts may be larger (I think mine were at least two cup sizes larger; they do go back to normal once you stop, to my husband's chagrin). Your stomach will still look several months pregnant (see my son's comment above). This is because your uterus takes about six weeks to go back to its prepregnancy size, and you've likely added pounds to help nourish the baby while in utero.

What about weight changes? I can only tell you my experience, but with each pregnancy, I gained 40 pounds (I'm pretty tall, five-foot, nine inches), and then lost about 12 pounds immediately after birth (with seven-to-eight-pound babies). I continued to lose another 10 or so pounds over the following month, probably due to loss of fluids. That put me at roughly 20 pounds over my prepregnancy weight. I eventually lost that weight without dieting, but it did take a full year for my first two babies (and I expect that pattern to repeat with this third).

How does breastfeeding play a role with weight loss? Yes, breastfeeding uses up a lot of calories, but you're also hungrier to compensate. One rule of thumb I've seen is to add an average of 500 extra calories per day if you're exclusively breastfeeding, 400 extra calories if you're mostly breastfeeding, 250 extra calories if you're partially breastfeeding, and zero extra calories if you're not breastfeeding. Personally, I have never felt comfortable dieting or restricting calories when breastfeeding because I don't want to affect my milk supply. This might be why it takes a year for my weight to go fully back to normal. Every person is different, and their journeys are as well. Give yourself and your body grace.

There are other symptoms that you might experience postpartum as well. These include heat flashes and night sweats those first few weeks after giving birth. I've woken up drenched in sweat several times. It can be annoying, but it will pass. Another symptom is hair loss. This symptom starts a few months after birth and peaks around four months. You're not actually losing that much hair, though it may seem like it. Your body didn't shed very much hair during pregnancy thanks to those hormones, so your postpartum body is basically going back to how your hair was prepregnancy. If you're worried, talk to your doctor about it.

Mental Health

Most women experience some baby blues. Your emotions are heightened for many reasons: it's a new experience (even with subsequent babies the experience is new) and your hormones change drastically. Estrogen and progesterone decrease, while oxytocin and prolactin increase. These changes happen very rapidly. You might cry and get upset more easily than usual. You may be irritable or even angry and not feel like yourself. But you've also just had a baby! It takes time to adjust, but if you're worried about what you're feeling, talk to your doctor.

How are the baby blues different from postpartum depression or postpartum anxiety? Postpartum depression and anxiety are much more extreme and last longer. One big red flag is having thoughts about harming yourself or your baby. If you feel yourself growing angry at your baby, set them down and walk away, even if they're crying. Go to a different room, cover your ears, and take a few deep breaths. Chances are you'll be okay going back in a few minutes, but you don't want to do anything rash. Seek help immediately if you're constantly overwhelmed or are experiencing extreme emotions or serious thoughts about harming yourself or your baby that don't go away.

Don't underestimate how refreshing it can be to get out of the house. Even a walk around the block can help. One of the ways I feel rejuvenated is by having lunch or coffee with a mom friend. Chances are she is going through (or has recently gone through) something similar, and talking about it and commiserating is therapeutic. If you're the first in your friend group to become a mom, try some online forums. Check out our Empowered Mama community on Facebook, where you can share your stories and gain insights from other moms. We're in it together!

In my opinion, sleep deprivation makes the hard days much harder. On days when I've had a decent (for the newborn stage) night's sleep, I am in a much better mood and can handle my screaming baby, toddler, and child more easily than if I've had a poor night's sleep. The importance of sleep may seem obvious, but it's useful to think about ahead of time because it can help you understand what you're feeling and why you may be quick to sadness or anger.

Finally, remember that it's brave to seek help. It can be hard to do, and sometimes there is fear and shame associated with asking. We all fight silent battles at some point, but we don't have to do it all alone. Taking time for yourself in whatever way you need will make you a better, happier mother.

There are also ways to get little wins. Thank your body for all it has done. A man's body couldn't do it; *your* body did. Practice gratitude if you can (e.g., "I'm grateful I got five minutes to drink my tea in peace today."). And finally, give yourself grace (e.g., "I made a mistake today, but I forgive myself. Tomorrow is a new day.").

Sleep

Speaking of sleep, try to get as much of it as possible. This is much easier said than done. If your baby is in a safe sleep space (or being held or watched by someone else), get some sleep. Maybe you didn't nap before having a baby. This needs to change now that the baby is here because chances are you won't be getting a full night's sleep (unless you are formula feeding and your partner or another adult is doing night feeds). I've been able to sleep sitting up and with the lights on, which under normal circumstances I would never be able to do.

If you are breastfeeding, consider having your spouse or partner sleep in a different room for the first few weeks. They will get a full night's sleep, and then they can take the baby during the day while you nap (provided they are taking time off from work).

There is more on this in the sleep chapter (chapter 4), but babies are very loud sleepers! Allow them their grunts, noises, and short cries. Don't rush to them because they may very well still be asleep or may drift off again if you let them. Waiting a full minute before you go to them is a good rule of thumb. If their cries are constant or increasing, then of course go to them to help them settle back down or feed them.

Because babies are loud, you might consider moving them to their own room (or at a minimum, to a distant corner of your room). While some people recommend waiting until six months or so before moving the baby to the nursery, we've never done this (even though I thought we would). We moved our first baby out of our room and into our nursery at about four to five months, our second at three months, and this one we moved out after four weeks. I have a monitor and can quickly get to them if needed, but the distance helps us both sleep better. The baby doesn't hear me and wake up, and I don't catch every grunt on the monitor the same way I would if he were right next to me. Turn your monitor's sound setting on a low level; you will still hear them crying, don't worry.

Asking for Help

This one was tough for me to accept, particularly with my first baby. I wanted to do it all myself and believed that I not only could but should. As a result, I was more tired and stressed than I needed to be. Asking for help doesn't mean you need to delegate the tasks you want to do. Be specific in what you need.

Do you want to shower and eat lunch in peace? Ask for someone to watch or hold the baby for half an hour. Do you want a solid two-hour nap? Ask for an adult to take the baby on a walk or simply hold them in the living room or watch them sleep on a safe sleep surface. On the other hand, does being away from your baby make you feel a bit anxious? I felt this way with my first, even if he was being held right next to me. So, ask for what you need. Can the person offering help do your dishes or laundry? Can they take your older kids for an outing or walk your dog? Can they bring you a home-cooked meal?

You might feel guilty about asking for something specific or asking for help with housework, but if that person truly wants to help you, they will. You are deserving of help, and it doesn't make you less of a mother to accept it. On the contrary, it will probably help ease your mental and physical load, and that will make you a better, more attentive caregiver to your child.

Sex

Will you ever be the same down there? There is hope! I have eventually felt back to "normal" a few months after each pregnancy. Doing Kegels can help you regain your strength, and sex becomes just as pleasurable again. That being said, it can take a while. For me, while I'm breast-feeding, I tend to have a much lower sex drive (even feeling asexual, with absolutely no interest, at times, though it has varied considerably with each postpartum period). Also, because of the hormones, your vagina doesn't provide as much natural lubrication, so lube is a must to make things less painful and more pleasurable, even if you didn't use it before. The first time you have sex postpartum can be scary, but try to relax and have fun with it, and as I said, use lube.

Breast and nipple play can be a huge turnoff if you're nursing, or maybe not. There's a huge range of "normal." I sometimes joke with my husband that my boobs are no longer his or even mine, but the baby's. Overall, the most important thing is to be honest and communicate your desires (or lack of desires). You'll want that communication to be a two-way street though. After all, your partner hasn't physically changed and wants to know that you still find them attractive and desirable. Compromise if possible and talk to your doctor if you're concerned.

Again, in my experience, my sex drive and vaginal lubrication return to normal once I'm done nursing. I'll also add that my sex drive has been different during each postpartum experience, sometimes greater and sometimes less so. Encourage out-of-the-bedroom foreplay (i.e., housework) from your partner. If you're not tired, have a clean house, have sleeping children, and feel appreciated, you're probably much more likely to be in the mood.

Fitness and Working Out Again

According to the Mayo Clinic, if you've had an uncomplicated birth and vaginal delivery, it's generally safe to start exercising again a few days after birth. When I read this, I immediately thought, "That was written by a man who has never pushed a seven-to-eight-pound baby out of their vagina." However, if I'm in a more forgiving mood, I might say they meant "exercise" that didn't refer to going on a jog or doing a plank. It could be as simple as climbing up the stairs or going on a walk around your neighborhood.

If you're wondering about when you're *really* cleared, I'd say two things: First, your OB-GYN can tell you if you're good to go during your postpartum appointment (about six weeks after birth). Second, your body will let you know when you're pushing too hard. If it's painful, stop. Pick something else that isn't so hard on your body. For example, exercises that require sharp movements to quickly change directions, like basketball or tennis, usually take much longer for me to do safely than things like swimming or cycling.

There are also really excellent resources for postpartum (and pregnancy) fitness. I find that the best option tends to be in-person if you can find it and with an instructor who has been postpartum herself. They empathize and can suggest movement modifications to help keep you safe. They can also make sure you're doing the movements correctly and give you feedback.

In lieu of in-person options, there are several online options that I like. For example, Materra Method has an app and website with plenty of classes that are rated for the stage of pregnancy or postpartum life you are in. Their founder, Abby Erker, is a pregnancy and postpartum exercise specialist, and this definitely comes through in her videos.

Motivation and finding time can also be frustrating factors. Just like pretty much everything else, working out changes after you have a baby. Whereas before you could dedicate an hour to working out and 15 minutes to shower and change, now, you likely can't (unless you enlist someone to watch your baby, and for me, I tend to prioritize other things when this happens). Celebrate the small wins. It's okay if you can only get four minutes in before your baby needs you again. Maybe you can do a bit more after you settle them back down, or you can give yourself grace and try again tomorrow.

Illness (Your Own)

I hate to break it to you, but you will get sick. And unlike before you had a baby, you are not allowed to be sick. That may seem a bit harsh, but I just want to prepare you. Your baby will not know or care that you are sick, and you will still need to care for them, wake up in the middle of the night with them, etc.

Slow down as much as you can and focus on caring for yourself and baby. Enlist help if you are able. Sleep and take medicine. Talk to your doctor about medicines if you're breastfeeding, though mine is always okay with the over-the-counter medicines I ask about. Interestingly, women tend to have stronger immune systems than men and don't get sick as often or for as long. Yet when it does happen, prioritize taking care of yourself, and you'll get better more quickly.

Working or Being a Stay-at-Home Mom

To quit or not to quit? If you were working before (and during) pregnancy, you may have asked yourself this question. I'm a working mom, and I have mom friends who are working moms and stay-at-home moms. Everyone seems pretty happy with their choice, though I know that decision isn't always a true, unconstrainted choice for some women (due to financial pressures or other considerations). I don't think there is a right or wrong choice. And, importantly, neither option is permanent. If you quit and decide you miss working, you can get another job. If you don't quit immediately, you can always do so later.

For me, this was a difficult decision. I didn't want to quit a job I enjoyed after I had spent so many years getting a postgraduate degree, but I also felt so emotional about leaving my baby. I was extremely lucky in that I was able to find a middle ground. I asked my (male) boss if I could go part time, to working 32 hours a week (every Friday off), and he agreed. I have remained on this schedule nearly five years later.

Some women work it out where they can work from home, but I don't recommend trying to parent and work at the same time. It just isn't feasible, and it's not fair to either your baby or work, as neither will get 100 percent of your focus. As someone who had an 18-month-old at home during the first few weeks of the pandemic, I can attest that it is an impossible task.

Some pros to continuing to work:

- Financial. Even with daycare or nanny costs as high as they are (and trust me, with three in daycare, I know how expensive it is), as long as you're making more money than you're paying for someone to care for your child, it's financially worth it. Plus, you will continue to gain skills, be on track for promotions, and build retirement savings, which will all help financially.
- Adult interaction. You will have daily adult interaction with people who don't just see you as a mother. Your conversations will be about more than diaper changes and how your kids are doing. You'll be able to eat lunch in peace.
- Appreciation. Motherhood is a thankless job, and that can make it even harder. At least at work you will hear that your output is appreciated (hopefully, if you have a good job).
- Balance. Doing something outside of mothering (which is fulfilling but very hard) and housework (which is mentally taxing and repetitive) can help you find balance. This doesn't have to be paid work. It can also be volunteering, doing something creative, or becoming involved in your child's school (related, but

not the same as mothering). You can also find this balance if you're a stay-at-home mom.

- Social interaction and intellectual stimulation for your baby. My son loves his friends at daycare, and I'm constantly surprised by how much he's learning (letters, writing, reading, science, math, etc.). I think these benefits are larger for kids who are two years and older; however, it does depend in part on the quality of your daycare.

Some cons to continuing to work:
- Less time with your baby. Little ones change so much that first year. You will miss some things, like their first word or first steps, and while you will likely see them repeat the milestone soon after it happened, it might not be the very first time they do it.
- Guilt. You may experience guilt about not being there all the time for your baby. I had a lot of guilt when pumping didn't work well for me and I had to supplement with formula. You won't be there for every boo-boo or to kiss them every time they are scared. You might feel guilt that your baby isn't getting food that you prepared yourself (though by the time they're three, they'll be so picky it won't matter). There is also a lot of emotional pain and guilt for you if your child gets hurt while at daycare (both my older kids have been bitten a few times).
- Fear that your baby will "forget" you. Some moms worry that their baby will prefer another adult. Indeed, this is one reason I preferred a daycare to a nanny. My kids have loved most of their teachers, and it's much better when they don't cry every time you drop them off. You're still the first person they turn to when you're there, don't worry.

Since I haven't been a stay-at-home mom, I won't speak to those pros and cons, though I imagine in large part they are mostly the flip of the pros and cons of continuing to work. Whatever your choice, your baby will love you. A happy mom equals a happy baby, so do what makes sense for you and your family.

Maternity Leave

If you do choose to continue working, you will hopefully be able to take some time off to bond with your baby. If you have a good job with benefits, you'll likely have some paid parental leave in addition to paid short-term leave. If you don't have these benefits but have been at your current job a minimum of a year, you'll at least have access to 12 weeks of unpaid time off through the Family and Medical Leave Act (FMLA). Your job will be legally protected for you when you return.

I had six weeks of short-term leave and six weeks of parental leave to be used within the first year after birth. With my first and second babies, I saved a few weeks in case they got sick (which they did). With my third, I decided to take the full time.

I usually have a to-do list a mile long for maternity leave. This time, it included things like finish our family's 2018 scrapbook, register the car, and plan a 10-year wedding anniversary vow renewal, my older kids' birthday parties, and my newborn's baptism. It did not include writing this book; that was added later! Your to-do list may be long, but if you accomplish one thing beyond keeping yourself and your baby alive, fed, clean, and rested each day, consider that a success. Don't stay up late to check things off your list. The time you have off is for bonding and resting, not for getting other things done.

7

Taking Care of a Newborn

"Sometimes the littlest things take up the most room in your heart."
—A. A. Milne, author of *Winnie-the-Pooh*

*N*ow that your baby has arrived, your main job is to take care of them! Unless you've nannied a newborn, you may be a little unsure of what the day-to-day will look like. This chapter touches on the main aspects of caring for a baby. A newborn care class (likely offered through your local hospital) is a good way to get some hands-on experience (with a doll) and is a place to ask questions. It may seem like there is a lot to think about and remember, and there is! But since you and your partner will be doing these things day in and day out, you'll become comfortable taking care of your newborn in no time.

Picking Baby Up

Picking up a baby was one of the things my husband was worried about before becoming a dad. Newborns seem so fragile! The most important thing here (other than not dropping them) is to support the baby's head. Those little neck muscles haven't had a chance to develop strength, so gently cradling their head with your hand is important. You can try holding their head with one hand and their back or bottom with the other. Then, you can hold the baby against your chest, over your shoulder, or on your arm.

Once you've picked up the baby, you can move them to your arms. You can hold your baby against your chest with one hand firmly against their back and the other arm's elbow tilting up to their head. Then, you slowly tilt them sideways until their head is in the crook of that arm, with their body supported by your forearm. You'll get the hang of it in no time. Dads in particular might like the football hold with the baby's head in the hand and body along that same arm and to the side of the adult's body. I find this hold a bit awkward as the baby feels heavier. Once your baby can hold their head up reliably, you can pick them up by their armpits. Do what feels natural and comfortable for you.

I've mentioned this elsewhere, but don't pick your baby up if you are angry with them. If you're holding your baby, put them down and step away briefly. It can really make a difference to your mood to step outside the room for a minute or two. Because of that lack of head control, it's very dangerous to a baby if you shake them, as their head (and brain) will snap back and forward. Keep your baby safe, always.

Tummy Time

Speaking of head control, your baby needs tummy time! Start with a few seconds (if they get fussy) and work your way up. My first and second babies really hated tummy time at first, but eventually they loved it and flipped onto their stomachs immediately (because they learned to crawl—freedom!).

Tummy time doesn't have to be done on the floor. You can place your baby face down on your chest or arm. Even placing your baby over your shoulder can be a good way to get them some practice. If your baby really doesn't like it, you can try a tummy time pillow or a rolled blanket under their arms. Moving their arms under their body and next to their head (elbows bent) can help a baby prop themselves up. Mirrors at eye level can motivate them, and so can you! Get down on the floor with your baby and smile and talk to them. When they get a bit stronger, you can position yourself on the other side of their head and talk, encouraging them to turn to face you! It's a great way to play with your newborn; just remember they tire quickly.

Car Seat Safety

You'll need a properly installed car seat to go home from the hospital. Go to a seat inspection place near you to make sure you have it installed correctly. You can use a seatbelt (great when traveling) or your car's latch system and the car seat base. Follow the manufacturer's instructions. Using the base makes an infant car seat easy to repeatedly get in and out of the car.

When your child is backward-facing, their head should be about an inch below the car seat's head rest. The shoulder straps should be below the shoulders. When you clip your baby in, make sure the chest clip is in line with their armpits (otherwise, if it's too high, they can choke, and if it's too low, they can slip out during a crash). You want to pull the strap to tighten it; pull on the chest clip to get rid of any slack around the shoulders and around the legs. You shouldn't be able to fit more than a finger under the shoulder straps, though there can be a little room around the hips. I recommend not using the provided shoulder pads (or pads you purchase). It can be hard to make sure the straps are tight enough with these pads.

Remember, your baby shouldn't wear a coat or bulky jacket while in the car seat. Even if you think you're tightening the straps, the bulkiness of the coat can make it impossible to properly secure your child. They could slip out or be injured in a crash. Instead, if it's cold, you can cover them with a blanket once they are buckled. You can also use a winter infant car seat cover, which creates a cocoon of warmth for them. Finally, if you do get into an accident, even a minor one, replace the car seat and the base. Not all damage is visible to the naked eye.

Diapering: Poop and More

Maybe you've never changed a baby's diaper before. You will. By the end of the first week, you'll be a pro. One of the most surprising things about a newborn's poops is that they are *loud*. Also, the poop can shoot out about a foot (or more), so try to get their little bum covered quickly by a clean diaper when changing them. My firstborn would poop all the time when he was being changed—on me, on the walls, on the stack of clean diapers, and on the furniture. He'd also pee everywhere, including on his own face, poor thing. My daughter never did and my second son has rarely done it, so in part it depends on your baby, but be prepared!

For boys, one perhaps shocking thing is that their penises get hard. That's right; they have erections. Obviously, it's not a sexual response and it goes away quickly, but this is why they can pee on their face. Sometimes baby boys will pee when you take the diaper off because of the colder air touching their bodies. To prevent this, you can try wiping just above the diaper *before* you take it off. The cold from the wipe can cause them to pee while the diaper is still on. There is a product for this called Pee-Pee Teepee, which is a tiny cloth cone of fabric that you can place on top of the penis during diaper changes. It's a funny idea, and it does work, though it's hard to keep it on if your baby moves around (which they will). Finally, it's also a good idea to gently point the penis down when putting on a new diaper. This way the pee is less likely to leak through.

Newborns need to learn how to poop! Relaxing the sphincter muscle takes practice and is difficult for them at first. This is why your baby will likely poop while they eat—they're relaxed. I often like to change my baby's diaper between breasts (or halfway through a bottle). I do this even if I think they might pee or poop at the end, and I know I'll need to change them again. Oftentimes it wakes the baby a little more and they get a full meal in, plus they feel nice and clean. You can drop this diaper change if they're getting full feeds in and just change them at the end. However, if at the end of a feeding you notice a small bit of the yellow indicator line on the diaper has turned blue (indicating they've peed a little), don't feel the need to wake your content baby up by changing their diaper. Diapers can handle a lot of moisture. Just think about when your baby eventually sleeps through the night; you won't be waking them to change them. The exception is poop; you'll want to change that immediately.

So, how do you actually change a diaper, and when should you? Almost all disposable diapers nowadays have a wetness indicator—a yellow, vertical line running up and down the diaper. It turns blue when wet. Because newborns need to eat so frequently (every two and a half to three hours, four to six hours at night if you're lucky), you don't usually need to check to see if they're wet. Simply change them after they eat (and in the middle of a feeding; see above). The exceptions are if they're very fussy, you might want to check to see if they need to be changed, and if you hear them poop, you'll want to change them. Stool left on the baby's bottom for too long can make the skin red and forms diaper rashes. If this happens, simply apply a layer of diaper cream (like Aquaphor or Desitin) to the area until it resolves.

It's easiest to change a diaper if you have everything close at hand. I like to place an open, clean diaper below the used one. This has saved me on multiple occasions if my newborn decides to pee or poop while I'm changing the dirty diaper. Make sure you keep a hand on your baby at all times. They might roll off a bed or changing table, even if you think they can't yet. You can change your baby on pretty much any flat surface—a changing table, bed, floor, even your legs while you're sitting (this is convenient when you're out and about).

Some diapers have "back" or "front" written on them, but if they don't, the back is the half with the tabs on it. Open the old diaper and use wipes if your baby has pooped. Then, remove the old diaper (you can put the dirty wipes inside), close it, and secure the tabs so the diapers and poop don't fall out. If you already have a new diaper under the old one, pull the top over your baby's genitals and secure the tabs. If not, place the clean diaper under the baby's bottom and do the same. The diaper should fit snugly but not too tightly. If you see red marks on your baby's upper thighs when you change them, it may be too tight.

Some diapers have a newborn cutout for the umbilical cord stump. If your brand doesn't, just fold the top down so that the stump can stay dry (see chapter 3 for umbilical cord care).

With a girl, it's important to wipe front to back to prevent bacteria from getting in her vulva and vagina. Carefully spread the vulva lips to get any poop that might be in those creases. For a boy, make sure to wipe under his scrotum (and over and around). Because newborn poop is usually pretty liquidy and yellow, it can blend into the skin. Run a wipe along the baby's crevices to make sure you get it all.

That brings me to poop frequency and color. For a newborn, the very first poop or two will be a blackish, sticky gunk known as meconium. After that, it will get yellower, more liquidy, and seedy. Formula-fed babies' poop is thicker and can be yellow-green or pale brown. Newborn poop really doesn't smell too bad and can have an almost sweet scent. My husband disagreed until our baby started eating "real" food. Then, the poop definitely stinks, so enjoy the newborn poop while it lasts. Colors can vary based on what you eat if you're nursing, but breastfed babies' poop is usually yellow. Colors to watch out for are black (after the meconium is done), white or a claylike color, and red. Call the pediatrician if your baby's poop is any of these colors.

As for frequency, a rule of thumb for the first five days is one poop and one pee per day of life (one on day one, two on day two, etc.). After that, there is a wide range of normal. Babies can poop every feeding or go a few days between poops. Breastfed babies poop more frequently than formula-fed babies. After six weeks or so, you might notice they poop less frequently. Their bowels are getting larger so they're able to go longer between poops. You will be asked to monitor your baby's pees and poops for the first few weeks and report on them at pediatrician appointments. It's a good idea to get an app on your phone to record this and make it easier to remember.

Finally, when should you size up on diapers? Different brands will be a little wider or longer, so while they will have recommended weights for the diaper size, you might find that a different size works better. My third baby was in the newborn size about three weeks, then size 1 for about three weeks, then size 2 (12 to 16 pounds in Huggies) when he was about 10 pounds. Sometimes they can be in between sizes for a few days and you'll be able to use two sizes. Smaller sizes are cheaper because they use less material and more fit in the package, but don't try to use them past when your baby truly fits in them. You can always donate unused diapers to a friend or churches (which often have diaper drives). If you're finding it hard to use the diaper tabs, then it's too small. If the diaper tabs have a significant amount of overlap, the diaper may be too big. Constantly having leaks (pee or poop) can mean the diaper is either too big or too small (I know, not very helpful) or that the brand isn't the best fit for your baby. You can pull out the frilly sides of the diaper around the legs to help hold poop in.

Packing the Diaper Bag

Packing the diaper bag isn't too difficult, but there are a surprising number of things to remember. Pack more diapers than you think you'll need. I suggest at least five at any given time. Include a pack of wipes (and switch it out when it's less than a quarter full), travel-sized diaper ointment, poop bags or a wet-dry bag, two full changes of weather-appropriate clothes, a muslin swaddle (it can be used as a blanket, changing pad, baby cover, or nursing cover in a pinch), hand sanitizer, a nursing cover, burp cloth, and extra pacifiers. I like to pack a hat and socks, travel-sized lotion, lip balm for me, and cash as well, just in case. Once they get older, you'll likely add toys and snacks (always pack snacks!). If you're bottle-feeding, you'll want to pack bottles, formula, and a water bottle full of water if you're mixing it while out.

Grooming: Bath Time and More

Bath time is fun but intimidating. Babies are very slippery when wet, so be careful. Before their umbilical cord falls off, don't submerge them. Lay out a towel to rest them on, and gently wipe the baby's body with a soft washcloth, warm water, and a tiny bit of baby soap. Don't get the umbilical cord wet at all. Make sure to wash in between all of their folds and creases and rinse off their body with warm water using a washcloth. I start with the neck and work my way down. Keep the part you're not working on covered so they stay warm. You can put a hat on your baby as well (most of the heat escapes from the head).

Finally, get a new washcloth and wipe the baby's eyes from inner to outer corner, using a new part of the washcloth for each eye. You can then do the baby's hair by squeezing warm water from the washcloth onto their scalp, gently rubbing a tiny bit of shampoo in circular motions with your fingers or a silicone baby brush, and then rinsing. It seems like a lot, but you really don't need to bathe your baby often. Some people say two to three times a week, but I bathed my third baby once a week, and that was enough. They don't really get dirty (blowouts being the exception).

After the umbilical cord falls off, you can submerge your baby's body! Don't dunk their head, obviously. Get the water to the right temperature and fill up the baby bathtub. Use the newborn sling until they can lift up their head securely. You could also use the tubs that go in the sink. Just make sure the water isn't flowing directly onto your baby and keep one hand or arm in the running water at all times (it can change temperature rapidly, and you don't want to accidentally burn them).

Either way (infant tub or sink tub), keep your baby's body covered with a soft washcloth and pour water over it every few seconds so it stays warm. Wash their body much like before, except now you can use running water. Remember, save their head for last; you don't want them to get cold too quickly. Also, fair warning: when a baby is nice and warm and relaxed in the bath, their sphincter muscles may relax, causing them to poop. Because of this, an ideal time for a bath is right after they have had a bowel movement.

Getting the baby out of the tub is intimidating. They're so slippery, and you have to juggle a towel! I often wait until my husband can help. One of us lifts up the baby and then hands it to the other person that has the towel to quickly wrap around them. If you're doing it yourself, the hooded towels are nice because you can clamp the hood part between your chin and chest, pick up your baby by securely grabbing them under both armpits, then pressing their back to your chest. Wrap one side of the towel over their body while keeping their body secure with your other hand tightly under their armpit or on their chest, then wrap the other side. You'll feel better after a bit of practice. If you don't feel comfortable with this method, you can lay the towel on the floor or counter, lift the baby up, and quickly move them to the towel.

Whatever method you choose, your baby may scream quite a lot when they are moved from the warm bath into the cold air. You can mitigate this a bit by moving quickly (but safely), prewarming their towel or their clothing using a heating pad, and putting a hat on your baby. Use lotion on them if you want and then put on their clothing.

Some books recommend giving an infant massage during this time. I've never found immediately after bath time to be optimal, however, given that they are pretty cold and upset. Instead, you could hold your baby chest to chest with a blanket on their back until they are warm, and then give them a massage if you want. This doesn't have to be long; just rub some lotion softly onto their body while singing or talking to them. Lotion is also really useful if your baby is a bit chubbier. My third had the most rolls, and I noticed the creases in between his little leg rolls would get red, almost like an open sore. Keeping the creases moisturized helps with this. You can also use Vaseline or Aquaphor or another petroleum jelly to be extra thorough.

There are a few more grooming-related points. Babies need their nails filed or trimmed. Their nails are quite soft at first, but they can be sharp. Since babies don't have good control over their limbs, they can scratch themselves, so you need to stay on top of this. I find infant nail scissors to be much easier than nail clippers. Some people also use a nail file instead. The easiest way to trim their nails is laying the baby on their back or having their back to your chest. This way, you can securely hold a finger and trim it much in the same way as you'd trim your own nails (the nails facing the same way as your own). I find I need to do this about once per week.

That perfect baby skin may suddenly look a bit more like a teenager's after two to four weeks. Infant acne is common, and it will go away on its own within a few weeks. Don't treat it; use only water on the face like you did before. Your baby's face will go back to that smooth perfection soon.

Around the same time, you may notice what looks like dandruff on their scalp. This is known as cradle cap, and it's common. It doesn't bother them, and you don't need to treat it. Don't pick at the scales. If you want to, you can rub a tiny bit of baby oil onto their scalp a few minutes before bath time, then use a baby comb to rub it out with shampoo using small circles. Some of the scales should lift off. You can also buy cradle cap shampoo. I've used Happy Cappy before. Be careful, though, sometimes you might pull off some of the baby's hair too. Hair loss isn't uncommon and peaks around four months. It may be more likely around the parts of your baby's head (like the back) that are rubbing on surfaces often. Don't worry; their hair will grow back.

Physical Development

It's shocking how quickly babies grow! You can almost see a difference day-to-day. My third baby gained nearly four inches and over five pounds in the first two months. Imagine growing that fast as an adult! When you go in for pediatrician visits, they mainly want to make sure your baby is gaining weight and staying at roughly the same percentiles as they were at birth. A baby's weight will double within four to six months and triple in the first year. Height gain will slow down, but a baby will still likely be about 10 inches taller than they were at birth by the time they celebrate their first birthday.

Newborns have many interesting instincts, all related to survival. They will grasp whatever touches their palms (palmar reflex), and their grip strength can hold their body weight for a second if using both hands (I don't recommend testing this). The rooting reflex helps them eat (they turn their head and open their mouth to a touch near their lips) as does the sucking reflex (instinctively sucking when something touches the roof of their mouth).

The startle reflex (or Moro reflex) is particularly adorable. When a baby is startled by a loud sound, or they feel like they are falling, they will shoot out their arms and legs, try to grab on, and pull their limbs back in. It's thought to give a caregiver an extra second to catch them if they fall (but again, don't test this). It's also the reflex that can wake them up, which is why swaddling is so important while they sleep.

Newborns also learn how to do a few things with their faces. They smile socially when they're around two months old, if not a bit sooner. A little later, they coo and "talk" to you, and a bit after that, they laugh (the best sound in the world). They can also be quite expressive with their eyebrows and mouths. They'll frown and pout when scared or upset, and they'll scrunch their eyebrows when concentrating (mine do this when they eat sometimes).

Interestingly, newborns don't cry tears until about two weeks old, sometimes longer. These won't be giant, fat tears like we have, but you will notice moisture at the corners of their eyes. Newborns also sneeze sometimes to clear out their tiny nasal passages. It's usually not a sign of illness unless accompanied by other symptoms.

Play Time

The first six weeks, a baby will do very little except eat and sleep. Then, they gradually become more alert and have longer periods of awake time. Of course, this happens after you finally think you have a bit of a routine (get used to this; your child will always be shaking things up).

Once they stay awake longer, it's a great idea to interact with them. At first, keep it simple. Newborns are nearsighted, and their eyesight is still developing. They see things best from 8-12 inches away, which is about the distance from your face to theirs while they are nursing. Newborns really like high-contrast images (black and white), and they like faces even more. In fact, psychologists have found that babies prefer an image of two squares above one square than the inverse, and researchers posit that it's because that image is more similar to a face. Talk to your baby and slowly move your face to the left or right. See if they can follow you with their eyes or head. If not, no worries, just keep practicing.

Newborns don't really need toys for the first three months. You can use objects found around the house, like a picture, a mirror, or anything high contrast. My babies were mesmerized by a pair of black pajama pants with white polka dots. I'd set them down and slowly walk by them, and they'd follow with their eyes.

If you do want to get some toys, play gyms are nice because you can set the baby on their back and they can reach for the toys. They really won't start doing this until around three months old though. I also like the NogginStik rattle. The base is black and white and has a mirror, and the top cycles through colors—blue, red, and green—that light up when shaken. My babies have all enjoyed following it with their eyes.

Play time should be pretty short at the newborn age—a few minutes at a time. You'll notice when they are done because they will look away, yawn, or even cry. They get overwhelmed easily, so don't push it. Your newborn is learning plenty just from your day-to-day routine. They will soon learn to play with all manner of toys, don't worry.

Language Development

The best time for a person to learn a language is when they are less than three years old. Think about it—do you really "teach" a baby to talk (with formal classes, online learning, etc.)? No, they pick it up as part of their natural development. You don't have to define every word; they simply get it from context and listening to those around them.

The same goes for a second (and third and fourth) language. I spoke Spanish to my first son almost exclusively for the first two years of his life. I remember hearing comments from others fearing that would delay his development of the English language. This is a common misconception. In reality, knowing a second language can be a great aid to your child. My son could say over 60 words by the time he was 18 months old (for context, about 10 words is more typical).

Since he turned two, it's been harder for me to keep up the Spanish. In part, it's because he would speak to me in English (because no one else understood his Spanish words) and I would naturally respond in the same language. And partly, it's because English is my default for more complex ideas. Unfortunately, now, at nearly five years old, his understanding of Spanish is less than I would have hoped, even with weekly Spanish classes. Immersion in the language is ideal, but you also need daily reinforcement. Even if you can't meet this intensity, I think exposure to another language has great benefits and no downsides.

Pediatrician

There are many pediatrician appointments in the first year. The first month alone you will probably see your pediatrician at least three times (a day or two after leaving the hospital, around one or two weeks, and at the one-month mark). At these checkups, you will be asked about your baby's behavior—are they eating well, are they peeing and pooping regularly, any concerns?

The first few checkups, you'll need to report how frequently your baby is eating (the number of times in a 24-hour period and length of time if nursing) and how much in ounces (if bottle-feeding). You'll also need to tell the nurse how many wet and dirty diapers they had in the last 24 hours. This is all easier to remember with an app (there are many free versions out there; mine is called Baby Tracker).

You'll also want to take a muslin swaddle or small blanket to these appointments to keep your baby warm because you will be asked to take your baby down to the diaper so that they can be weighed and examined. A baby might lose some weight in the first few days after birth, but by the two-week mark, they should have gained it back. They grow a lot (see physical development section in this chapter), but don't worry too much about percentiles. Your doctor is mainly concerned that they are gaining weight and that their percentiles stay roughly similar to what they were before. They'll also check to see how tummy time is going and how the baby's head control is developing.

Write down anything that concerns you leading up to your baby's appointment and take the list with you (keeping it on your phone is the easiest). That way you don't forget anything once you're there. You never know what could be abnormal. For example, my first baby always liked looking to the left. He frequently turned his head that way and would immediately turn it to the left if we turned his head to the center or right. He had mild torticollis, a condition in which the neck muscles contract, causing the head to twist to one side. The solution was to gently turn his head to the right and hold it there a few times a day, but it could have gotten worse if we didn't mention it.

I also remember asking about a pulsing I saw on my baby's soft spot on the top of his head. I was worried it was his brain swelling! Turns out, it was completely normal and was just the blood pulsing (corresponding to his heartbeat). Had I not asked though, I wouldn't have known. Talk to your pediatrician about anything that worries you regarding your child.

Illness

Unfortunately, your baby will eventually get sick. Their immune system is not fully developed yet, and they haven't received vaccinations (the first round is usually at the two-month visit, and then it takes two weeks for those to kick in). Illness in newborns is thus scary and dangerous. This is why it's so important to restrict visitors and touching when babies are very young. A fever over 100.4 degrees those first three months is a medical emergency. Take your baby to the emergency room and call their pediatrician. By the way, the most reliable way to take a newborn's temperature is through a rectal thermometer. Buy one that is newborn specific (the tip is very short so you don't go in too far). Turn on the thermometer, use a glob of petroleum jelly on the tip, lift and bend your baby's legs (like you'd do for a diaper change), gently insert the thermometer into the rectum and wait for it to beep, indicating the reading has been taken. Clean the thermometer afterward with hot water and soap.

Some signs your baby may be sick include:

- Loss of appetite (not eating as frequently or not as much)
- Change in pees (especially very few or no pees)
- Change in poops (fecal matter with a lot of mucus in it)
- Vomiting (this is different from spitting up; for example, vomiting green bile)
- Fever over 100.4 or low body temperature
- Coughing regularly
- Floppy limbs
- Change in body color (e.g., turning bluish)

If your baby is struggling to breathe or wheezing, this is not normal and you should call your pediatrician. If their crying sounds different (e.g., weak, hoarse, or otherwise strange) that could be a sign of illness as well.

Basically, when in doubt, call your pediatrician. It's better to be safe than sorry. I remember as a first-time mom, I didn't want to be "that mom"—the one who would freak out at every little thing and unnecessarily bring her baby in. When my son was two months old, he was extra fussy and coughing a lot. That day, I nursed him in the shower to help calm him and help him breathe. The next day, we took him to the pediatrician. His oxygen level was lower than they liked, and they sent us to the emergency room. He had respiratory syncytial virus (RSV) and bronchiolitis from the RSV. He needed to be hospitalized and put on oxygen for two nights. It was very scary, and I was kicking myself for not having taken him in the day before.

The bottom line: trust your motherly instinct.

When it comes to medicine, ask your baby's pediatrician. Acetaminophen (e.g., Tylenol) can usually be given early on, whereas ibuprofen (e.g., Advil, Motrin) cannot be given until a baby is at least six months old. Your pediatrician should be able to give you a sheet with dosage based on weight. Keep a copy right by the medicine so you don't have to search for it when your baby is sick. My philosophy with these pain and fever reducers is to not overmedicate but also to give them when I think it's necessary, especially if the baby's fever is creeping up.

A quick story: One warm April day, my 19-month-old simply started seizing. It was the most terrified I'd ever been in my life. We rushed to the hospital in an ambulance (this was April of 2020, meaning early COVID-19 era, so all our neighbors were home and quite curious). My son had a seizure because his temperature rose too quickly and his little body couldn't handle it. The fever wasn't uncommonly high (103 degrees Fahrenheit), but the speed with which it rose caused the seizure, called a febrile seizure. It's never happened again and didn't cause adverse consequences, but now I'm quick to give Tylenol or Advil (to an older child) when they have a fever, and I make sure to retake their temperature frequently. Again, call your pediatrician when in doubt and listen to your motherly instinct.

Finally, to end on a much less scary note, make sure you give your baby vitamin D drops (made for infants) if they are primarily breastfeeding. You should do this daily from the time you get home from the hospital, so it's a good idea to have some on hand before you go into labor. The packaging will tell you the correct dosage (you need 400 international units; in some brands, that is just a drop, while in others it's more than that). Vitamin D helps newborns absorb calcium and phosphorous, and since they shouldn't get direct sun exposure at this age, supplements are necessary. Breast milk is awesome, but it doesn't provide enough vitamin D. Formula includes it in high enough doses, so if you primarily formula feed, your baby won't need the supplement.

A Day in the (Newborn) Life

You'll likely quickly fall into a loose daily routine. Your baby will slowly start to have more awake periods, and this is a really good time to interact with them! You can read to them or sing to them, and their favorite "toy" right now will be your face. My eight-week-old lights up when I smile about a foot away from his face and talk or sing to him. He's also started cooing (an "oooh oooh" sound). Tummy time can be hard to fit in at first because babies sleep so much and you don't want to put them on their bellies too soon after eating. Soon, though, you'll be able to do more of it, and they will likely grow to enjoy it!

Much of your day will be filled with eating, sleeping, and changing the baby (see chapter 4 on sleep for an hourly schedule). I recommend occasionally getting out of the house too, even if it's just a walk around the block, and chatting with other adults, particularly moms of young kids. This can help keep you balanced. And while you may have a to-do list, don't forget to just enjoy your baby and document the passing time. I like to take a picture of my baby lying on a small, elephant-shaped blanket each morning. I did this for my first two kids every day of their lives for the first year (even on vacations). It's really amazing to see them grow up day by day. You'll hear this more times than you can count, but time really does fly (even if a single difficult day can seem never-ending ☺).

8

Newborn Must-Haves

"All you have to do is love them. That's the only thing they need."

—my mom

*N*ewborns need very little. As long as they are warm, dry, and fed, their needs are 95 percent covered. Your face and voice are enough to entertain them for a long time. However, I'm sure you're wondering what else could come in handy and what you should put on your registry. Below is a list of things that have been helpful to me in the first few months, along with recommendations and a list of don't-needs. Most of the items are useful during the newborn phase, though I added in a few, like stair gates, that are useful a few months after that.

These recommendations are all based on my own experience and were current as of the time of publishing this book. Make sure you do your own research, and check for recalls because things can change quickly in the baby world. None of the product recommendations were sponsored or given to me for free. They're simply what has worked well for my family. Ultimately, your lifestyle and personality will influence what you want for your baby, so have fun putting your own list together!

Absolutely Need

A few of these categories are so important that they have their own chapters or major sections in a chapter! Check them out if you want more information.

- Diapers. We considered cloth diapers (there are services that pick up soiled diapers and launder them), but ultimately given that the cost and environmental impact were similar to disposable diapers because of the energy needed to launder them, we went with disposable. I've tried several brands (see Diaper Dabbler if you want a sample pack), including various bamboo brands and the two big ones: Pampers and Huggies. Ultimately, I think what works best depends partly on your baby (torso length, thigh size, propensity for blowouts, etc.). My oldest primarily used Bambo Nature (bamboo), my second Andy Pandy (bamboo), and my newborn is currently in Huggies Little Snugglers. Andy Pandy would be my bamboo recommendation (over Bambo Nature and DYPER). I like Huggies, though, because they don't have a smell (some Pampers do), they're fairly economical, and they have a poop pocket (so do some Pampers), preventing blowouts up the back. I have found that they're better at containing messes than Andy Pandy. Use what works best for you. I'd get two jumbo packs in the newborn size (newborns go through roughly 20 diapers a day, so that should be enough for about two and a half weeks). My third baby had moved up to size 1 diapers by the end of week three, and he was in size 2 by week seven. You can get more diapers pretty fast, so two jumbo packs should be plenty. If your baby is measuring big at your final ultrasound, you may want to have some size 1 diapers on hand as well.

- Wipes. Use what works for you. I like WaterWipes and Pampers Aqua Pure. Basically, the fewer ingredients, the better. I honestly think high-quality wipes are a main reason my babies have not had severe diaper rash. Overall, I like WaterWipes more as a wipe, but the Pampers Aqua Pure container seals better and the wipes are interlocking, making them more convenient when trying to pull several out.

- Clothes. I suggest long-sleeve footies with a zipper because they are very easy and prevent you from needing other types of clothes, like socks or hand mittens. I suggest five in the newborn size and five to ten in the 0–3-month size (sometimes known just as 3-month). See chapter 9 about clothing for more specifics.

- Vitamin D drops (if you're primarily breastfeeding). Breastfed babies need these administered every day. Start as soon as you bring your baby home from the hospital. You can buy vitamin D drops that come with a syringe and the kind that is just one drop a day. The one with a syringe is a bit annoying because you have to clean it every day, but the one drop a day one can be frustrating if you miss slightly. (Did they get the full dose in?) Choose whichever type works better for you.

- Car seat. Don't buy this used. I recommend an infant car seat, which people sometimes call a bucket seat. Even though some convertible car seats can grow with your baby from birth, the infant car seat can be transferred to a stroller, carried on errands or into your house. This is very convenient if your baby falls asleep in the car; just make sure to keep an eye on them—sleeping on their back is the safest! It's worth investing in a good car seat because they can be used for seven years. My third child is using the infant car seat his older brother used nearly five years ago. I have an UPPAbaby Mesa car seat. This brand is on the pricier side, but I think it looks very nice and the stroller combo is great. Also, a mouse chewed through the fabric while it was in storage, and the company sent a replacement for free, even though it had been three years since we purchased it.

- Crib. Like a car seat, don't buy this used because you never know if it was recalled or if it's still safe or not. Most cribs will have three different heights that you can adjust to have your mattress high (newborn age, easy access), medium (rolling over, sitting up), or low (standing up). Again, invest in a good one because your child will be using this for years. Side note—do *not* take your toddler out of their crib or convert it to a toddler bed until you absolutely must. Once they're no longer caged (ahem, I mean, contained) in their cribs, your nights and early mornings can include a surprise visit from your toddler. Plus, you know they're not getting into anything unsafe while you think they're asleep. Consider a GREENGUARD Gold certified crib, which means it's free of nasty chemicals. Some cribs will tout being three-in-one or four-in-one, meaning they go from crib to toddler bed (railing with a small opening where they can climb down) to daybed or twin bed using attachments that are either included or purchased separately. It seems nice in theory, but we've only ever gotten to the toddler bed stage before buying a different product. I got a Natart crib. The construction is very solid. I also purchased a cheaper crib for my toddler once my third baby was born, and the back was fairly flimsy. See the crib in a store if you can to check out the quality.

- Crib mattress. If you have a crib, you need a mattress designed for an infant. This basically means it is very firm. Some have springs (which I don't recommend), some have waterproof covers (very nice to have; it wipes down in case of spit up, a potty accident, or throw up), and some are dual-sided, meaning that one side is firm (for the first nine months or so) and the other is a bit softer (for a toddler). Some mattresses even tout being "breathable" in case your baby turns face down. Crib mattresses aren't cheap, but this is one area where I recommend making sure what you purchase is high-quality. I have purchased some that were not too expensive, but I ended up returning them because they simply felt uncomfortable (e.g., Dream on Me). All my kids have slept on Moonlight Slumber Little Dreamer mattresses. They're GREENGUARD Gold certified, waterproof, and dual-sided; I really like this mattress.
- Crib sheets. Make sure you get ones that will fit your mattress. I suggest buying at least three in case of overnight messes.

- Swaddles. See the section on swaddles in chapter 4 on sleep. You will want at least three swaddles. They keep your newborn from startling themselves awake and function as a blanket to keep them warm while they sleep (real blankets are a no-no at this age during sleep according to safe sleep guidelines).
- Nail scissors or nail file. I find baby nail scissors to be much easier to use than nail clippers. Use a nail file if you're worried about cutting their fingers.
- Baby soap and shampoo. Babies don't need much more than water to keep them clean. Most baby soaps are a soap and shampoo combination. Use whichever brand you prefer; Johnson & Johnson and Dove are widely available. Pretty much all of the baby brands that I have seen are paraben free.
- Rectal thermometer. You'll want one that is specifically designed for a newborn. A rectal thermometer is the most reliable way to take their temperature at very young ages.

Nearly Necessary

This list is the longest because, as I said before, newborns need very little. But there are many products that make your life a bit easier, and in those first few months, many of these items become an indispensable part of your routine.

- Bassinet. If you want your baby to room-in with you for a while once you get home from the hospital, you may want a bassinet. You can use a crib instead, but bassinets are smaller and easier to fit in your room. We had a HALO swivel bassinet I liked with my first baby. By the second though, we had caved and gotten a Snoo. Snoos are the very expensive Rolls-Royces of bassinets. They have built-in white noise and rock your baby in a side-to-side motion all night long. Both the white noise and the motion automatically increase up to four times with your baby's cries. If your baby is soothed, it gradually lowers back to the baseline level. At the highest level, it will time out after about a minute so that you can step in because your baby needs you. I swear by our Snoo, and we take it with us even when we travel those first three months. The weaning off process isn't bad (there is a setting for it). You can rent it if you prefer, and they offer military and other discounts.

- Bassinet sheets. Buy the ones specific to your bassinet; you want a tight fit. I'd get at least three. One tip I read long ago was to double up on your sheets, that is, from the mattress up, put on a waterproof sheet, then a regular sheet, then a waterproof sheet, then a final regular sheet. That way, if your baby pees through a layer, you just have to peel that off. It makes things a bit easier in the middle of the night. However, if your mattress is waterproof, this isn't really necessary.

- Monitor. When your baby eventually moves to their own room, it's nice to be able to see and hear them without having to go into the room. I've been through five or six different kinds of monitors. My favorite is the Miku. You install it on the wall above the baby's crib, and it monitors their breathing if you have a subscription (without any attachments on the crib or baby, like other brands). It's expensive, but I really like it. It also works through Wi-Fi, which is convenient to use later on when you get a babysitter because you can check in on them if you're a bit nervous leaving your baby (like I was the first few times, though honestly, I still always check in). It's expensive but worth it in my opinion. You don't need a subscription for it to work when you're in the same house, but if you want to check in when you're not on the same Wi-Fi, or if you want access to the breathing features, you'll need a subscription. VTech is also an impressive brand, with many reasonable options, a great picture, and good-sized monitor screen (depending on which one you get). We use this when we travel. I've also used the monitors from Infant Optics and VAVA. Both were fine, but I like Miku and VTech better (better features and monitor, respectively).

- Bottles and formula. This moves to the absolutely need category if you're not breastfeeding. It's generally a good idea to have some on hand before your baby is born just in case breastfeeding doesn't work out for you (by choice or otherwise). See the section in chapter 5 for bottle and formula suggestions.

- White noise machine. This one can *almost* go in the absolutely need category. It helps your baby sleep (see chapter 4 on sleep), and anything that does that is critical. We like the Hatch Rest for when we're at home and the Dreamegg for when we're away from home. You can download a white noise app on your phone in a pinch, but it does drain your battery and then you have to leave your phone close to the baby.

- Baby bathtub. A baby bathtub with a newborn sling is incredibly convenient to bathe your baby. I first had one of those giant flowers that go in the sink, but those were hard to dry, and it got moldy quickly. Now, I have a Puj Flyte, which is the same idea (goes in the sink), but the material is nonabsorbent. It folds in half so it's very easy to travel with. I also have one of those plastic tubs that has an infant size and a toddler size, as well as a newborn sling. These are very nice too, particularly when the baby can sit up by themselves. In addition, we have an inflatable duck bathtub. It's bigger than the plastic baby tubs so it works great through about two years old, plus it travels well. We also have an Otteroo, which looks like an inflatable float ring except it's tiny, and it goes around the baby's neck. That might seem concerning, but it doesn't choke them. My babies really seem to enjoy it because they can float and feel very lightweight. You use it in an adult-sized bathtub so pressure isn't put on their necks.

- Diaper bag. Any bag will do, just make sure it has lots of pockets. You'll want to fit diapers (at least five at any one time), wipes, one to two extra changes of clothes, a blanket or traditional swaddle, burp cloths, nursing cover, diaper ointment, and hand sanitizer. I like the chic Itzy Ritzy mini, but you may want a larger bag initially. Regardless of the one you choose, you'll likely have to replace it within a year or two because it will get near-daily use.

- Breast pump. If you're going back to work, this becomes an absolutely need unless you are the rare mom whose baby is in a daycare in the same building where she works. Even then, there will likely be times you need or want to pump. My favorite pump is the Elvie Pump. It's quiet and wireless. You can wear it in your nursing bra and be hands-free. You could also rent a hospital-grade pump (more intense sucking), but with today's technology, I don't think it's necessary (and they're incredibly bulky). I've used a Spectra S2 as well, and while it was fine, the Elvie is much more convenient.

- Baby carrier. There are free-form wraps and then more structured kinds of baby carriers. I have both types. I find that the structured kind is nicer when your baby get bigger because it offers more back support and more evenly distributes the weight. I own three carriers. One is a Boba wrap, which is nice if your baby is lighter than eight pounds, though that stage doesn't last long. It can, of course, be used when they are older as well. My favorite for the newborn age through about six months old is the Boppy carrier (they must be over eight pounds). It's a little like a structured wrap. I also have a LÍLLÉbaby carrier, which is convenient when they get heavier.

- Stroller. There are so many strollers out there! I have three kinds, and I like them all for different purposes. My main stroller for going on errands, out to dinner, or on pavement is the UPPAbaby Vista. It's expensive, but it looks nice, goes with my car seat, and has aged well these past five years. It also has various attachment options for if and when your family grows. There is a bassinet for when your baby is a newborn (though honestly, I haven't used it with my third baby at all), an infant car seat attachment, two different sized seats for when kids are older, and a standing board you can attach as well. In total, that means that up to three kids can use it at a time. Other brands offer similar configurations. Use what makes the most sense for your budget and your style. The second type of stroller I have is a jogging stroller. This is great for babies who are six months or older. The wheels are bigger and in a triangle shape, with one in front and two in back, making jogging with a baby easier for them in terms of bumps. Even if you don't jog, you might want to consider one for off-pavement purposes, like walking on a dirt path. Finally, I have a travel stroller. I've tried four brands, and my favorite is the Summer Infant 3DPac CS+. It's a trifold stroller, meaning instead of folding in two, it folds into thirds, making it extremely compact (like a cube, sort of). It's perfect for car or plane travel (we took two to London with our two older kids), and it's also very convenient to throw in the back of your car as a "just in case" stroller.

- Diaper rash ointment. You can avoid most diaper rashes by using quality diapers and wipes and by keeping your baby's bottom dry by changing them frequently (especially poops). However, chances are your baby will have a diaper rash at some point. I really like Aquaphor (you don't have to buy the baby-specific one). I keep a small tube in the diaper bag and one in the nursery. It's also multipurpose (think dry skin, chapped lips, etc.). For tougher diaper rashes, I like Desitin.

- Burp cloths. Your baby may spit up a lot or very little. Either way, when it does happen, it's nice to have a soft burp cloth to catch or clean up the mess. I'd have at least 10 and closer to 20 on hand. You may go through several a day.

- Pacifier. Some people may not want to use pacifiers, but babies need nonnutritive sucking (see chapter 4's "Soothing Tricks" section). It calms them. With my first baby, my boob basically provided this, which was not fun and made it difficult to tell when he was truly hungry versus just wanted to suck. I recommend the newborn Tommee Tippee pacifier.

- Tylenol. This is good to have on hand, though make sure to use it only after your pediatrician has okayed it. That being said, use Tylenol when your baby needs it (e.g., after shots, teething, fever, or when generally sick and miserable). Note that Children's Tylenol and Infants' Tylenol have the same strength, 160 mg/5 ml, so they are interchangeable. Infants' Tylenol *used* to be more concentrated, but not anymore.[3] Don't believe me? Check the label! The infant version has a nice syringe, but once you have that syringe, you can buy Children's Tylenol, which tends to be cheaper. Don't use Infants' Advil or Motrin until after your baby is at least six months old. Infants' Advil or Motrin *does* have to be Infant, not Children—different strengths.

- Lotion. Some people swear by infant massage, but none of my babies has liked it. I use lotion every few days after a bath to help keep their skin from drying out.

- Snot sucker. Your baby will get sick at some point, and their tiny noses will get stuffy and runny. It's hard for them to get that snot out, and it can make it tough to breathe. The hospital will likely send you home with a bulb syringe, but I don't find these particularly effective or sanitary. We like the NoseFrida. In fact, I swear by it. It's basically a plastic chamber connected to a mouthpiece by a tube. You put one end on the baby's nose, the other to your mouth, suck, and the baby's boogers come out. Does it sound totally gross? Yup. Will it become indispensable when your baby

---

3   Selena Simmons-Duffin, "Tylenol for Infants and Children Is the Same. Why Does 1 Cost 3 Times More?" *NPR*, May 27, 2019, https://www.npr.org/sections/health-shots/2019/05/27/726327937/tylenol-for-infants-and-children-is-the-same-why-does-1-cost-3-times-more.

is sick? Also yup. We keep one in the diaper bag and always have one when we travel. At least it's better than the alternative—my older coworker talked about doing it the old-fashioned way—no tools other than your own mouth. Yuck!

- Baby hairbrush. I have a super soft baby hairbrush and one that has a fine-tooth comb as well as little silicone nubs that are good for gently scrubbing the baby's scalp to help with cradle cap.
- Blankets. You'll want a couple small baby blankets of varying thicknesses. Your baby will eventually need one if they go to day-care (for naps after they turn a year old), and if you have a winter baby, you'll need a few to cover them up when you go out.
- Baby washcloths. It's good to have several of these on hand for bath time. Baby washcloths are softer than your typical towel and quite small.
- Hats. I rarely use them, but I do find having a newborn hat or two nice, particularly when getting them out of the bath (most of their body heat escapes through their head). I'd also suggest having some hats in larger sizes. Babies outgrow the newborn size quickly. If you have a winter baby, you should probably invest in a few more extra-warm hats.
- Stair gates. Get one for every staircase. You won't need them in the newborn phase, but babies will learn how to climb stairs sooner than you think. They won't know the dangers, so keep them safe!
- High chair. This is one of those products where there is an unbelievable number of brands that make them, without much difference between the options. Mine is a Peg Perego, which offers lots of recline options, a big tray, and a compact fold. I suggest getting a high chair that has various recline positions; that way, you can use it from a very early age. There are also high chair options that attach directly to the table. These are a fun concept, but I've never used mine much.

Nice to Have

- Rocking chair or recliner (or combination). Get one that is extremely comfortable; you'll be using it often.
- Breastfeeding pillow. These are very convenient if you're nursing. I like My Brest Friend for when the baby is a newborn because it is sturdy and supportive. It has back support as well. The Boppy pillow is nice when your baby is older and heavier, and it can double as a place to prop your baby up or to use for tummy time when they're bigger.
- Heating pad. I turn it on and place it on the swaddle in the bassinet when I pick up my baby to feed him at night. I think this makes the transition back to the bassinet easier for him because it's warm. As a bonus, you can use the heating pad on your back during labor (this really helped me) and postpartum in case your back is sore.
- Humidifier. I've gone through several and really like the Vicks brand. The baby version has a nightlight, it's simple to operate, and you can add a Vicks pad to help open your baby's congested nasal passages.
- Diaper pail. We have a Munchkin diaper pail. Actually, we have two, though we usually just use the one. You don't technically need one, and baby poops aren't too smelly before they start eating real food. However, given the number of diapers you'll go through, it's nice to have what amounts to a big trash can that looks somewhat nice to contain them. Don't forget liners.
- Car mirror. A baby needs to be backward-facing in their car seat for as long as possible (my 22-month-old is still backward-facing), so a car mirror is really nice to have in order to see them while driving. It gives some peace of mind; for example, if they're crying or screaming, you can see if they're really okay, or if you might need to pull over.

- Baby chest rub. This can be used on babies that are at least three months old. I think the smell is soothing and may help them breathe more easily when they're sick. Vicks BabyRub or Zarbee's Baby Chest Rub are two brands I like.
- Bottle sterilizer. When you're a first-time parent, you worry a lot more about the bottles and pacifiers being perfectly sterilized. It's nice to have the first few months, but as long as you do a good job cleaning them and use hot water (hand washing or in the dishwasher), I think it's okay to not sterilize every time when the baby's a bit older.
- Baby detergent. Dreft laundry detergent is responsible for that baby smell. Seriously. The reason this isn't in the nearly necessary category is because I don't think you necessarily need baby-specific detergent. If your family already uses a hypoallergenic one, then great. If not, make the switch. A baby's skin is so sensitive those first few months; you don't want them to break out in a rash because they have a reaction to their clothes. Make it easy on yourself and wash the whole family's clothes in the same hypoallergenic detergent. After all, your clothes will also come in contact with your baby's skin.
- Saline nose spray. This helps dislodge those tough-to-get boogers.
- Memories and milestones blanket, book, signs, etc. Your baby will grow so much the first year, and even though it may feel never-ending in the moment, it really will go by quickly. To help you document this time, I suggest getting a milestone blanket (Etsy has good options) and a book (I like *Baby's First Year: A Simple Book of Firsts*). You can also do hand and foot prints. I did these in plaster around two months and every three months with nontoxic ink. I've continued doing their hand and foot prints at more infrequent intervals with each child, and it's pretty amazing to see the growth for my nearly five-year-old!

- Baby lounger. We have three of these. It's very convenient to have one in each of your most used rooms (we have one in the kitchen and one in the bathroom, which is great for cooking and showers, respectively). We have a BabyBjörn, a lounger that came with our pack and play, and a Boppy newborn lounger (which was recalled for being unsafe for sleep, but I keep it because it's great for posing newborns for photos and I never let my baby sleep in it). I don't think the brand matters too much here; just pick one or two that work for you.
- Stroller fan. If you have a summer baby, a stroller fan helps keep them cool. They're inexpensive and clip or wrap around the stroller.
- Winter car seat cover. Because you should not buckle your child in their car seat while they are wearing a winter coat, a car seat cover is very convenient during the cold months. It's sort of like a cross between a thick blanket and a coat that goes outside the infant car seat. It has a little cover you can open for them to breathe better, but you can close it when you go outside briefly in the cold air.
- Age-appropriate books. I love reading and hope my kids will too, but newborns need you talking to them more than the books themselves. If you want to get some that your younger infant will enjoy, think simple, high-contrast pictures (black and white, for example) or a book of faces. For older infants, one of my favorite series is the *Never Touch a... (Dragon, Shark, Polar Bear, etc.)*.
- Warming breast pads. This can help with your let-down or help with engorgement. I like the reusable kind that you microwave to warm.
- Nipple cream. I like Earth Mama Nipple Butter, which you don't have to rub off before nursing.
- Diaper caddy. It's convenient to store diapers, diaper ointment, wipes, and lotions in this, but it's not truly necessary.

- Changing table pad. These usually have raised sides to keep your baby from rolling off, though of course you should always be right next to your baby (and touching them) while changing them. We have a regular one and the Hatch one. The one by Hatch wipes down easily and is also a scale.
- Waterproof changing pads. I like to have at least 10 of these on hand. They're small and have a waterproof backing, so they're very convenient when your baby has a blowout or pees while changing them. You can just throw it in the wash instead of whatever is beneath it (e.g., sheets, couch cushion).
- Pacifier sanitizer. We have one made by Munchkin. It's convenient if your baby's pacifier or tiny toy falls on the floor and you don't have access to water and soap, or you don't have a spare— always have a spare!
- Pacifier wipes. Similarly to the sanitizer above, these wipes clean fallen pacifiers and toys. They use baking soda, which means they're food safe. I still wash the toy or pacifier with soap and water when I have access to it, but the wipes are useful in a pinch.
- Poop bags. These are sort of like the ones for a dog. They do make poop bags for babies though, which have odor-suppressing capabilities. These are nice when your baby poops while you're away from home (and don't want to or can't throw the diaper in a trash can), or when your baby has a blowout. You can contain the clothes in these until they can be washed.
- Wet-dry bag. This is the reusable version of the above poop bags. When the mess isn't too bad, I use this instead. I also have one that I use for my wet pump parts.
- Baby bum wand. This is convenient to apply diaper ointment so that your hands don't get sticky.
- Nursing cover. To nurse in public, you could use a blanket or swaddle, but nursing covers offer 360-degree discretion and are convenient. I have a WeeSprout cover that is nice and big, and I

caved with my second child and got the expensive The Cocoon, which is breathable and can be used as a shawl or scarf. Nursing covers can also be used as an infant car seat cover.

- Supportive seat. This is a seat that supports your baby as they learn to sit up. It's nice for when your baby can support their head but can't sit by themselves yet, and once they can sit, it keeps them contained so that you can feed them. Bumbo is a popular brand, though I like Upseat because it doubles as a booster seat at the table. My daughter used hers until she was almost two (she eventually refused to sit in it because she wanted to be like the rest of the family and sit on the big chair, despite almost not being able to see over the edge of the table).
- Activity mat. Also known as a baby play gym. Once they are a bit older (two-plus months), babies may like to interact with these mats, which usually have cute characters they can reach toward when on their back. These are much more useful after the fourth trimester, a.k.a. the end of the third month.
- Car seat blowout protector. I only had to use this for my first baby because he would consistently have blowouts in his car seat. It was nice to only have to throw the protector in the wash and not disassemble the car seat's cover to throw in as well.
- Infant gas drops. I didn't use these with my first two, but my third baby sometimes seemed to have gas troubles. I honestly don't know if it helped that much or not, but it made me feel better to use.
- Clothes hamper. Babies can use yours, but it's nice to keep their (poopy) clothes separate, and having one in their room is convenient.
- Walker (push kind). This is the kind of walker where they just stand and push. My older son loved his, but you won't use one for the first eight months (at least). Just be careful around stairs.

- Outlet covers. My kids have never shown any inclination to stick dangerous things in outlets. They have, however, tried to plug electrical plugs in or have tried taking them out. Outlet covers are a good purchase, and if you have something you need to keep plugged in that can't be covered by a piece of furniture, they also sell covers that allow plugs to be used.
- Baby spoons. You won't need these until your baby starts solids at four to six months, but they're nice to have once you do.
- Baby towel. The ones with the hoods are especially useful, and their small size is convenient so you don't have to constantly be doing big towel loads of laundry.
- Baby hangers. These are usually velvet and pretty small (to fit baby clothes, of course). It's convenient to have a pack on hand for those special outfits, though I think drawers are easier for everyday clothes.

Don't Need

- Changing table. We actually don't have a changing table. When my baby sleeps in the same room as us, I change him on our bed, and when he is in the nursery, we simply have a changing table pad on top of the dresser (which I secured with double-sided carpet tape). The dresser looks nicer than a changing table, in my opinion, and it can be used for years, not just months.
- Wipe warmer. I had one with my first child, and it ultimately wasn't worth it. The wipes dried out, especially near the end of the package, and the heat and water from the warmer created a crack in the dresser upon which it sat. Your baby will be just fine without a warm wipe.
- Bottle warmer. If you need to warm a bottle, you can simply put hot water in a mug or bowl and place the bottle in it for a few minutes to warm up. If you're primarily bottle-feeding, a bottle warmer may make more sense for you, but for me, it was

just an extra appliance. Also, your baby will drink whatever they are used to. I have friends whose babies drank breast milk or formula straight out of the refrigerator or at room temperature. Be warned, if you always warm up the bottle for them, they may *only* accept it warmed, which can be a hassle when you're traveling or running errands.

- Tummy time pillow. This is a small, C-shaped pillow used to prop up a baby for tummy time. I have one and it's nice, but a rolled-up blanket would work as well.

- Head pillow with cutout. These newborn pillows are marketed to help prevent a flat head, but in my experience, they are not necessary. Unless you keep your baby lying on their back all day and they don't turn their head to the side, you'll probably be okay without one.

- Baby swing. This is a step up from a baby lounger; it's basically the same thing but it moves, usually electronically. My friend swore by hers (a MamaRoo), but my first two kids didn't like it, and while my third does, I don't really think it's necessary. If your child doesn't like it, your baby swing basically ends up becoming an expensive baby lounger.

- Walker (sit and roll). Don't buy the kind of walker where your child sits in a seat in the middle and rolls around; these are dangerous (e.g., child rolling down the stairs and getting injured).

- Pack and play. If you have a crib, you really don't need a pack and play. If you stay at hotels when you travel, they will provide a crib or pack and play. However, if you stay with someone or at an Airbnb, then you will likely want to bring one.

- DockATot. We bought a DockATot because it was so popular, but honestly, I have been disappointed. Your baby shouldn't sleep unsupervised in it, and they can only lay on their back in it, so it's basically an expensive blanket with raised sides.

- Owlet Smart Sock (and the like). You wrap this "sock" around your baby's foot, and it tracks their oxygen and heart rate. At first glance, this seems really awesome. I'm sure it could be, but I have one and haven't used it more than twice. For us, it's just an extra hassle that isn't necessary. Many parents report false alarms, which could be pretty scary; I can't comment on that since I haven't used it much, but I'd imagine that would be very frustrating.
- Baby mittens. I purchased some for my first baby but ended up not using them. Just stay on top of keeping your baby's nails trimmed and you'll be fine.
- Baby mobile. I have a mobile that has black-and-white, high-contrast images as well as more complex images you can change out as the baby grows older. I don't think having one is necessary, though your baby may like looking at the pictures occasionally.

Don't Need Until After 12 Months

- Stuffed animals. This one's at the very top of this list for a reason. Babies don't care about "stuffies," as my four-year-old calls them, until they're at least two, in my experience. We have approximately 300 stuffed animals. People love to buy them as gifts, but there are only so many that your child can play with, you can't always donate them, and they take up a huge amount of space. Plus, chances are your child will have their few favorites, and everything else will simply accumulate dust. Buy a few now if you must, but wait until they're a toddler to buy more.
- Baby shoes. If you want them for photo ops, great. However, your baby won't need shoes until they actually start walking. In fact, some shoes can be bad for their walking development. When you do need shoes, I like the Stride Rite brand. Their Soft Motion shoes are built for those first steps. They come in half sizes and have options for babies with wide feet.

- Step stool. A baby won't need a step stool the first year. Their balance won't be great yet and you don't want to encourage falls by having one accessible to them.
- Pillow. Newborns shouldn't use a pillow to sleep (nothing should be in their crib except for them and a tightly wrapped swaddle). They don't need a pillow for a very long time. My nearly two-year-old still doesn't have one.

9

Dress-Up Time: Baby Edition

"Always have a change of clothes. Otherwise, you might find yourself wrapping your baby in the shirt off your back."

—Me, from experience

*T*here are so many cute baby clothes out there! Unfortunately, babies will outgrow them very quickly, and when the babies are older, the clothes will easily get stained (sometimes after just one use! Why do toddlers use their shirts as napkins?). Because of this, it's not worth spending a lot of money on expensive clothes.

I suggest having a cute take-home outfit in the newborn size. In general, opt for comfort—think soft fabric, zippers whenever possible, and large necks if you have to pull it over their head (you don't want to do this too often with a floppy-headed baby, trust me). Lots of newborn and infant clothes will have a neck that makes it easy to go over the baby's head or down their body. This is especially useful for blowouts.

I suggest long-sleeve, zippered sleepers for most of their clothes the first two months or so (sleep gowns are nice for overnight). You don't have to worry that they're cold, and you won't have to worry about finding pants or socks and keeping them on. Many zippered sleepers have a flap you can pull over your baby's hands, so you won't need baby mittens either (I don't think they're worth it anyway; just keep their nails filed or trimmed). You may want a few cuter outfits for milestone pictures and some plain ones you won't mind keeping tucked in the diaper bag just in case.

Bow headbands or soft clips are great for girls. They look adorable and prevent strangers from calling your daughter a "he," which never bothered me but might annoy you.

Because babies outgrow or ruin clothes quickly, I suggest going on the cheaper side when possible. Walmart (Wonder Nation) and Target (Cloud Island) have really cute baby clothes. Both carry Gerber outfits too, which have colorful patterns and offer some nice basics. Etsy is great for personalized outfits. Beware of shopping online at a retailer like Amazon. Some of the clothes from oddly named brands may appear cute and reasonably priced but have odd sizing, questionable fabrics, and poor durability.

You might also try your local baby and child resale store. I've had great luck with these. You can get name-brand clothing at clearance prices, and usually they're in pretty good shape because these places don't accept torn or stained clothes. Also, because kids outgrow clothes very quickly, the pieces are usually not too worn out.

If you want some nicer outfits, I suggest waiting for a sale and then thinking about the future (e.g., buying a Christmas or Easter outfit during a Labor Day sale). Some of my favorite brands for expensive but nice clothes include Janie and Jack (fancy outfits), Magnetic Me (magnetic clasps instead of buttons or zippers), Bums & Roses (cute patterns, bamboo clothes), and Kissy Kissy (soft sleepers). Mott50, Caden Lane, and Hanna Andersson are good brands for family-matching swimsuits, and Caden Lane, Hanna Andersson, and Ivy City Co. have family-matching outfits.

Infant Sizes

Infant sizing can be confusing at first. There's the newborn size but also 0–3 months; isn't that the same thing? No, it's not. Newborn size is usually up to about eight or nine pounds, so bigger babies may not even use this size at all. I'd suggest having a few newborn outfits for the first month and more in the 0–3 size. You might also see the 3-month size instead of 0–3 month. This is the same thing. When the size only has one month on it, you can think of that as the last month. So, 6-month would be the same as 3–6-month, and so forth.

My babies have all followed clothes sizing fairly consistently with their actual age. However, don't try to force your big baby to wear their smaller "age-appropriate" clothes and vice versa. Some brands run large or small. For example, my kids have to stop using Kissy Kissy clothes about a month before other brands (my kids are all tall). If you're shopping at Carter's, compare the size to another outfit. I remember buying a size 18–24-month pair of shorts that my son wasn't able to use until he was three years old. Meanwhile, other size 18–24 Carter's shorts fit fine. This sizing inconsistency has happened multiple times with this brand, so beware.

What Clothes Do I Need? Newborn Edition

When picking newborn clothes, strive for comfort. Here's a suggested list of the basics. You may want fewer or more of certain clothes to suit your style, how frequently you do laundry, and your baby's propensity for blowouts.

- 3 to 5 bodysuits, size newborn and 0–3
- 3 to 5 pants, size newborn and 0–3
- 5 sleepers or footies, size newborn
- 5 to 10 sleepers or footies, size 0–3
- 2 hats, size 0–6 (hats usually have a larger range)
- 1 pack of socks, size 0–3
- 1 to 2 zip-up hoodies (for colder months)
- 1 winter bodysuit (for colder months)
- 1 sun hat or swim hat (for summer babies)
- 1 going home outfit from the hospital, size newborn (not necessary but nice to have)

- 1 to 3 extra cute or fancy outfits, size 0–3 (great for milestone pictures or special events)
- 1 pack of bows if you have a girl (the stretchy headband kind are great at the newborn age)

Washing Clothes

You can wash your baby's clothes in any hypoallergenic, gentle detergent. It doesn't have to be baby specific. I suggest washing the whole family's clothes in it (after all, your baby's skin will touch your clothing too). However, if you do want a detergent specific for baby, I suggest Dreft—it gives the clothes that "baby smell."

Tags and the Plastic Part

The best brands know to make clothes tag-free. I'm always shocked by brands that have three-inch, scratchy tags in baby clothes. I prefer to cut these big tags off so that they don't bother my baby. When you first buy clothing, make sure to cut the plastic tag holder (called a Garvey tag, who knew?) and discard both parts. I like to hold the part on the inside of the outfit while I cut it. This way it doesn't get lost. The last thing you want is for it to poke your baby and bother them. They can't tell you what's wrong, so don't let it happen!

Sun Care

Infants are not supposed to use sunscreen until they are at least six months old. But your newborn can and should be outside. So, how do you protect them? Keep them covered up or in the shade whenever possible. Use SPF-rated clothing if you're going to the pool or beach as well as a hat.

10

Outings and Travel

Can you get out and about with a newborn? Yes! Not only can you, but you *should* leave the house for your own sanity. That being said, there are some precautions you should take (and things you should pack).

If possible, limit certain excursions and longer trips until your baby's immune system is more developed and their first round of vaccines has had time to kick in (around two and a half to three months). If relatives are dying to meet your baby, encourage them to come to you instead. If you do decide to travel, try to limit exposure. Think back to COVID-19 days—eating outside at restaurants, keeping your baby in their infant car seat and covered if you're somewhere indoors, limiting plane travel to more necessary trips, etc. Don't let people touch your baby. You can say something like, "We're not letting people touch him while he's this little."

Some easier trip examples include going on a walk (yes, this counts), a car ride to get snow cones, or sitting outside at your favorite breakfast restaurant. For shorter trips, you just need to pack the diaper bag (see the "Packing the Diaper Bag" section in chapter 7). Pack more diapers than you think you'll need.

Car Trips

Longer trips are possible too, but you need to consider a big question. Are you comfortable hearing your baby scream? They could cry during your entire car trip. At young ages especially, hearing my baby scream is hard on me. With my third baby, we went to my in-laws' lake house for the Fourth of July. It's only an hour drive, but with 20 minutes left, both my toddler and my newborn started crying. I couldn't take it and pulled over. Now, when we leave the house, my husband drives and I sit squished between the two car seats in the back. I can comfort my toddler and put a pacifier in my newborn's mouth. It's physically uncomfortable for me but works much better for my mental state.

Longer car trips can also be stressful in terms of needing to pull over to nurse or bottle-feed your baby. If you need to warm a bottle or access running water, it can be more difficult to do so during a car trip. It's not impossible—they sell portable bottle warmers and you can stop at a gas station for running or bottled water—but it is more complicated than when you're at home.

The nice thing about car travel is you can pack a lot of bulky items that will make your trip easier (e.g., baby's bassinet or pack and play, nursing pillow, large pack of diapers). However, unless you have a baby that reliably sleeps in the car, I'd avoid long car trips until your baby is old enough to be entertained. If you do decide to go, make sure to schedule extra stops along your route.

Train Travel

Taking the train is a little easier than the car in that you can walk around, feed baby, and hold them. Of course, you'll probably have to take a car to your final destination. That being said, the train is fairly convenient. You may still want to wait a few months for your baby's immune system to develop given that you'll be sharing the train car with others.

You won't be able to pack as much for a train as you will in a car, and keep in mind that unless your destination is the final one, you will only have about five minutes to get yourself, your baby, and your personal belongings (including car seat, stroller, suitcase(s), etc.) off the train before it starts moving again. Having another adult there to help you is ideal.

Plane Travel

You can get on a plane with your newborn. As with other trips though, you want to take their age into account. Waiting until they're at least two and a half to three months old is better. Additionally, be aware that plane travel is much more complex with a baby than it is without one. You'll have to navigate at least two airports, crowd onto a plane, survive the plane ride, and deplane. Your baby will be breathing in recycled air on the plane, and no doubt at least one passenger will be sick.

You'll have to lug around a stroller and a car seat. Yes, you can rent a car seat from a rental car company, but these are not infant car seats and they can be tricky to install (you'll have to do that yourself).

The good news is that a baby flies free. They do need a ticket though. Check with your airline because with some you get the baby's ticket the day of the flight at the ticketing counter, while with others you have to do it online beforehand. However, if you want to take your infant's car seat in the cabin of the plane, they will need their own (full-price) seat. I recommend this because it's nice to have the extra space and it's safer for your baby to be buckled in.

Packing for a Longer Trip

Yes, I know I've said that babies don't need a lot, and while this is mostly true, there are a surprising number of things you'll likely want with you when you travel for the sake of comfort and convenience. Depending on your method of transportation, you may be limited in what you can take.

Taking a pack and play or your bassinet may not be possible if you take a plane or train, and your baby's sleep may suffer for it. Cribs at hotels are not nice. There, I said it. Some are very overused pack and plays. Others are technically cribs, but their safety seems questionable. The mattresses can be overly thin or not have a fitted sheet (some hotels only provide a regular twin or queen sheet that you have to tuck under the mattress).

Taking a car seat is also bulky, and if you're on a plane, you have to pay for a seat unless you check the car seat (and I don't recommend doing this because it will likely get dirty or banged up). Diapers take up a lot of room. You can buy them at your final destination, but they may not have your brand or size, and you'd have to make an extra stop for them.

Certain things you've gotten used to, like a nursing pillow, rocking chair, changing table, and diaper pail, will be hard or impossible to take with you. There are also several things you may need to take but might not think about. For example, if you're bottle-feeding and going on an extended trip, you'll need dish soap. You might also want to consider bringing laundry detergent if you'll be gone for a week or more and are particular about the detergent used to launder your baby's clothes.

Here are a few additional things you may want to bring on an extended trip:

- A white noise machine
- More clothes than you think your baby will need (I pack double the amount of days we'll be gone).
- Sun protection
- A baby carrier
- A monitor if you're going to be sleeping in a separate room from your baby
- A travel stroller (like a trifold one, which folds down compactly into a thin, square shape)
- Your baby's medicines and vitamin D drops
- Tylenol and a snot sucker like the NoseFrida, in case your baby gets sick

All that being said, it really is possible to travel with your baby! Just be aware that you won't have access to the same conveniences and setup you have at home. Travel is enriching, but where (and when) you decide to go is largely based on your comfort with discomfort. Getting away from your typical routine can be energizing, but build in time to recover after the trip if possible. I've never felt like I needed a vacation more than after I'd just been on a "vacation" with kids.

Church

If you attended church prior to having a baby, you may be wondering what it's like after your baby is born, and if and when you should return. I'm Catholic, so my answer is going to be based off that experience, though I'm sure it generalizes somewhat. It's actually fairly easy to take a newborn baby to church. They sleep a lot and can be soothed when holding, rocking, or feeding. It's much harder to go to church when they are toddlers.

Go if you're comfortable. I'm much less likely to take my babies during the winter months when people are sick and coughing. You might consider watching a mass or service online instead. If you want to go physically, there are oftentimes cry rooms, which are separate and have toys (this is good when they're a bit older, around the toddler stage). Some churches even offer daycare during services so you can drop off your baby or child and actually pay attention, which is great.

Another thing: I often feel so guilty about not attending church after a baby is born. Interestingly though, the Catechism of the Catholic Church paragraph 2181 states:

"The Sunday Eucharist is the foundation and confirmation of all Christian practice. For this reason the faithful are obliged to participate in the Eucharist on days of obligation, unless excused for a serious reason (for example, illness, the care of infants) or dispensed by their own pastor. Those who deliberately fail in this obligation commit a grave sin."

I never knew this until my third baby. Since a baby is considered an infant from zero to 12 months, this knowledge lifted a weight from my shoulders and made me feel loads better. Everyone's spirituality and religiosity vary, and you can always talk to your pastor or priest about your concerns.

11

Dad, Siblings, and Pets

"Parenthood is the highest highs and the lowest lows."
—Matt, my husband and father of three

Dads

Your world changes greatly when you have your first baby, and your baby's dad's world does too. For them, it might even be a greater shock at the beginning. I remember my husband saying it didn't really hit him until he held our son in his arms (and the baby pooped on him). I think this is because while mothers have had nine months of physical and emotional change preparing us for a baby, Dad has not. You've literally felt your baby kick you and move around constantly those past few months. Because of this, remember that you and your partner *both* need time to adjust.[4] My husband has said that he doesn't truly bond with the baby until they are more mobile and can play. From what I've read, this is common among fathers; they tend to bond through play.

You're going through a lot postpartum and are experiencing things that are new to you and that your partner may be unaware of. Communicate these changes and your feelings. It can be helpful if Dad reads up on the postpartum period and how to take care of a newborn (chapters 6 and 7). That way, he knows a bit more on what to expect and how to help you.

---

4   While this section is written to apply to dads, parts of it could just as easily apply to a mother that did not give birth to her baby or to another adult partner.

My husband is a wonderful father and partner. When it comes to parenting newborns, however, he often lets me take the lead. You might think that you and your partner are going to be equal parents. I believe that is possible, but there *are* gender differences. I've experienced these—as have all of my mom friends, no matter how equal their partnerships. If there is a primary parent, more likely than not, that will be you. You'll probably spend more time with your baby, either because your parental leave is longer or because you become a stay-at-home mom. Dad will likely take cues for the baby's care from you and sometimes be unsure what to do. While you may also be unsure, you'll probably act first to take care of your baby's needs.

Then, there are all the hormonal changes you're going through. If you're breastfeeding, oxytocin will be released in your brain and your baby's brain too. That will help you bond with your baby. Dad doesn't get this benefit to the same extent, though he does get some oxytocin from holding and playing with the baby. To encourage Dad to bond with the baby, leave them alone for an hour while you get a pedicure, go on a walk, pick up dinner, or just go to a different room and watch an uninterrupted TV show.

An additional gender difference: women are impacted more by a baby's cry. Remember when I said I couldn't stand to hear my baby cry in the car? (See chapter 10 on excursions and travel.) My husband lasts much longer than I can. When we sleep trained our first child (12 months in!), I couldn't handle it and had to take a shower or leave the house. There's science to back this up.[5] A study found that when women heard an infant crying, their brain patterns zeroed in on it, they were more likely to feel sympathy than men were, and they were more likely to want (I say need) to care for the infant. In other words, when you hear your baby in distress (i.e., crying), you're in distress too.

This isn't true in the same way for dads. It's not that they don't care; they just don't have the same biological reaction. Moms are literally

---

5   "De Pisapia, Nicola, et al. "Sex differences in directional brain responses to infant hunger cries." *Neuroreport* 24.3 (2013): 142-146.

wired for a baby's survival. Keeping this in mind can bring a level of perspective and understanding when your baby is crying in the middle of the night and Dad is fast asleep. Communicate (during the day, especially). Ask Dad to take a turn; he may not know that you've already been up three times in the middle of the night dealing with the baby.

One thing my mother told me before I had my first baby was that my relationship with my husband would change. I accepted this but also sort of disregarded it. He was the love of my life; that wouldn't change. And it hasn't. However, in a lot of ways, my kids have come first (before myself as well). This is especially true when they are newborns and if you are breastfeeding. Your baby relies on you at least every three hours to survive. That makes it difficult to have quality one-on-one time with your partner.

Additionally, you may not have sex for a while—most doctors recommend waiting at least six weeks after birth or until the lochia stops. You might wait longer because you're simply not ready or because you're not sexually aroused like you used to be. This is especially likely if you're breastfeeding (see the "Sex" section in chapter 6). That being said, men's desire has probably not changed (even if you're feeling self-conscious about your changed body and less than sexy). What's important here is open communication. Tell him what you want and need. For example, if he helps a lot with your baby, you may have more energy and desire to be with him physically.

Something else to be wary about is becoming roommates with your spouse or partner. I think this is more common when there are multiple kids and little free time, but it can happen with just one child as well. Becoming roommates is when you live together but aren't really *together*. You each contribute to the household and childcare (hopefully), but it's a tit-for-tat, transactional relationship. To counteract this, make time for one another that isn't baby related. Do something together while the baby is asleep. When they're a little older, you can leave your baby with a grandparent, trusted friend, or babysitter, even for an hour, and reconnect with your partner. It makes a big difference. You will make it through the infant phase; make sure your relationship does too.

Siblings

This book is primarily written for women who are about to have their first baby. However, you might be planning ahead and wondering how things will look different with a second or third child. In terms of pregnancy and the newborn phase, you'll probably be ready to fill your own book! But how will your firstborn react?

My son was almost three years old when I had my daughter. I was worried that he would be very jealous. Instead, it was shocking how quickly he adjusted and how loving he was (and still is). Then, when I had my third baby, I worried that my much younger daughter (about 20 months) would be jealous. She was certainly more jealous than my son, but she has also handled it well. She's mostly a helpful toddler and has only tried to hit the baby a few times(!).

Siblings ultimately adjust. Yes, they frustrate and challenge each other, but primarily, they love each other. Before I had a second child, an experienced mother told me one of the most wonderful things was seeing the kids interact. I thought that was a strange thing to say, but now I get it. I see it when my eldest son takes my daughter by the hand as they're walking, or when she wraps her little legs around him when he picks her up. Or when both older kids rush to find the baby's pacifier or beg to hold him. It's heartwarming. However, when they do get jealous, make sure the older kids know you still love them and value your time with them. Try to have some quality one-on-one time with your older kids whenever possible. And let them be kids; they're not an additional parent or caretaker and shouldn't be treated as one.

It's also hard as a parent to go from one child to two (or three). My first maternity leave, my husband and I watched two TV series, napped, and had evenings together. By the third maternity leave, we were playing hot potato trying to juggle three kids and had almost no free time. I've heard (and corroborated through my own experience) that going from zero to one is harder on Mom, one to two is harder on Dad (each adult has a child), and two to three is a chaotic juggling act. You learn to let things slide more with each subsequent child and become a more relaxed parent. It's all a balance.

In terms of spacing children, I think three years was easier than the 20-month gap. My older son knew when to be quiet and could be briefly entertained by a TV show if I needed to put the baby to sleep or otherwise was unable to immediately attend to him. I think if I were a stay-at-home mom, the close age gap would be even more difficult. That being said, every mom and family is different. We adapt as moms, survive, and even thrive! Moms are everyday superheroes, truly.

Pets

Finally, a brief section on pets. My husband and I had two dogs before my first child. They were five years old by the time my first was born, and we loved them. We took them on trips, they frequently slept in our beds, and once we even had a birthday party for them where we invited their dog friends over and had a dog-friendly cake in the shape of a bone.

Once our son was born, our priorities shifted greatly. Our baby didn't sleep well, and I didn't have extra energy for myself, let alone the dogs. One dog would hide in the darkest corner she could find in the basement because she was depressed. I sometimes wore the dog on my back in a doggie carrier with the baby strapped to my chest to help the dog through her depression!

The whole family adjusted, and the dogs are happier now, but they do realize they are below the kids on the hierarchy. Watch your dogs (and cats and other pets) closely when around the baby. You never know if and when an animal will snap out. If it's a cat, you have to worry about them tracking bacteria from the kitty litter. My dogs have a nasty habit of eating poop, so I make sure they don't lick my kids' faces or hands.

Families adjust and the kids bond with the dogs (or other pets), which is really cute. But if your pet has a hard time adjusting to a baby or a handsy toddler, consider hiring a dog trainer to help, or for extreme cases, rehoming your pet for the safety of your baby.

The Quick and Dirty Summary

*P*regnancy is hard but also miraculous. Rest, slow down, and enjoy your kid-free time while you can!

Once your baby comes, ask for and accept help, even if it's difficult. Remember to take care of yourself—your family will be happier for it.

Newborns need very little: just your face and voice for entertainment, clean clothes (I suggest many zip-up, long-sleeve sleepers/footie pajamas), diapers, and breast milk or formula. A baby carrier and stroller are very helpful. Babies only need about one bath each week unless they get dirty. Keep up with your baby's pediatrician appointments.

Do tummy time when you can. Try to establish a good feeding schedule (every three hours) that's flexible when it needs to be. Avoid letting your baby "snack"—eating for short periods of time (five minutes or less) for comfort. They are probably fussy for other reasons, most likely sleep (a baby can be overtired, making it harder for them to sleep and causing them to mimic hungry behavior), gas discomfort, or being overstimulated. Separate feeding from sleep by promoting a little awake time after they eat. In other words, try to avoid feeding them to sleep.

Sleep when your baby sleeps (easier said than done), and always put them in a safe sleep space if you're sleeping yourself. The more they sleep in this way, the easier it will be. It may take some shushing or patting from you, or picking them up multiple times, but ultimately it pays off. White noise is key! Importantly, if your baby isn't crying (truly crying, not just making grunts or other noises), leave them alone! This gives them a chance to self-soothe and go back to sleep. When the baby does cry, wait a few seconds before going to them and try to soothe without feeding unless it's been at least three hours between nursing sessions.

Make time for your partner. Hire a cleaning person if you can or make peace with a dirtier house, send laundry out to be done by a business or family or friends looking to help, don't cook elaborate meals, eat off paper plates, etc. Basically, prioritize your baby, your other kids, yourself, and your partner. The rest can wait.

Try to limit interactions and travel until your baby's first immunizations. Have visitors wash their hands, and don't let them in if they're sick (people can be horribly obtuse about this). It's okay (and good) to leave your house with your baby—just keep them covered up and don't be afraid to kindly but firmly ask people not to touch your baby (people are also way too friendly with a newborn baby). Sit outside at restaurants if possible.

Relax and enjoy this time. It can sometimes seem impossible when you're sleep-deprived, but the newborn phase will soon pass. If you're feeling overwhelmed, very sad, or angry, leave the room for a few minutes (yes, even if your baby is crying), pass the baby to someone else for half an hour, take a shower or a walk, and breathe. If your symptoms are extreme or last longer than you think they should, talk to someone—a trusted mom friend especially (partners are great, but they don't have the same hormones and experiences as you do)—and your physician or a therapist.

Give yourself grace. I'll say it again—give yourself grace. You won't be perfect, but you are perfect for your baby. You're what they need, and you can do it. As my husband said once, "Parenthood is the highest highs and the lowest lows." It's a humbling and wondrous time. Good luck, mama. You've got this.

—Ana

About the Author

I'm a mother. I will never attach "just" to that title, as I've heard some of my friends (particularly stay-at-home moms) do. No one is just a mother. First, you're a whole person, with likes, desires, and dreams outside of motherhood. Second, motherhood is *hard*. It's a full-time and underappreciated job. It has value, not just to your family, but to society (see this blog post I wrote for my other job, the one I'm paid to do[6]).

So, yes, I am a mother—a mom to three wonderful children, ages four, one, and one month. I'm also many other things. I have a PhD in social psychology and am currently working at the Federal Reserve Bank of St. Louis as a senior researcher looking at economic disparities, like the racial and gender wealth gaps). I don't have any formal training that has helped me write this book (other than a few developmental psychology courses). What I mostly relied on are my own experiences as a mother. That, and the fact that I wrote this book during maternity leave, right in the thick of newborn bliss and sleep deprivation. I think that gives me, and this book, a unique perspective. There is a lot you forget once you're out of the postpartum and newborn phase. Writing about it now will hopefully give you some tips to help you prepare.

Other than my paid and unpaid jobs, who am I? Well, I love to try new restaurants and foods. I love to travel, particularly internationally (that has been harder, though not impossible, with kids). I also really enjoy reading, mostly fiction (check out books by Sarah J. Maas if you need a maternity leave reading list). I'm a planner—I love to plan trips, parties, activities, you name it! I'm also a sports fan, though I really only like watching games live (my alma mater, the Notre Dame Fighting Irish, or the St. Louis Blues). Finally, I'd consider myself to be artsy. In my paid job, I'm very analytical—writing scripts in statistical software to solve quantitative problems. But in my home life, I like to

---

6   Ana Hernández Kent, "Why Supporting Working Moms Benefits Families, Employers, and You," Fed Communities, August 8, 2022, https://fedcommunities.org/benefits-supporting-working-moms.

exercise the other side of my brain. I like to paint and do ceramics, and I play the violin (though I practice much too infrequently). I am also now only three years behind in my annual scrapbooking labor of love.

Mostly, I'm just a person trying to love my spouse fiercely, raise my kids well, enjoy my life, be there for my friends, and generally be a good person. I don't meet these goals every day, or even every week, probably! But I do try, and I think oftentimes the joy is in that daily attempt.

Thank you for reading this book. I hope it helps you enjoy your babies and your motherhood journey. Join us on the Facebook community Empowered Mama if you'd like to connect with me and other moms experiencing the same things as you. I wish you the best.

—Ana

Join the
Empowered Mama Community

What's your story? Have a question or a suggestion? I'd love to hear from you, and other moms would too. Join our Facebook group, Empowered Mama, and share your experience, get personalized tips, and connect with other moms going through the same things.